GLOBAL
TIME
BOMB

JOHN M. DORRANCE

GLOBAL TIME BOMB

THE COMING H3N2v VARIANT
SWINE FLU PANDEMIC
AND OTHER GLOBAL HEALTH THREATS

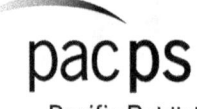

pac ps

Pacific Publishing Studio

Published in the United States by Pacific Publishing Studio

ISBN-13: 978-1469910215

ISBN-10: 1469910217

Special acknowledgement is made to the following:
Content Research: CDC.gov, PandemicFlu.gov
Cover Photography: Lorelyn Medina, Donetskaya Donetsk, BigStock Photo, iStock Photo

TABLE OF CONTENTS

1

A Global Pandemic

Though remarkable advances have been made in science and medicine during the past century, we are constantly reminded that we live in a universe of viruses and bacteria that are forever changing and adapting themselves to the human host and the defenses that humans create.

Influenza viruses are known for their resilience and adaptability. While science has been able to develop highly effective vaccines and treatments for many infectious diseases that threaten public health, acquiring these tools is an ongoing challenge with the influenza virus. Changes in the genetic makeup of the virus require us to develop new vaccines on an annual basis and forecast which strains are likely to predominate. As a result, and despite annual vaccinations, the U.S. faces a burden of influenza that results in approximately 36,000 deaths and more than 200,000 hospitalizations each year. In addition to this human toll, influenza is annually responsible for a total cost of over $10 billion in the U.S alone.

A pandemic, or worldwide outbreak of a new influenza virus, could dwarf this impact by overwhelming our health and medical capabilities, potentially resulting in hundreds of thousands of deaths, millions of hospitalizations, and hundreds of billions of dollars in direct and indirect costs. A pandemic is a global disease outbreak. A flu pandemic occurs when a new influenza virus emerges for which people have little or no immunity, and for which there is no vaccine. The disease spreads easily from person-to-person, causing serious illness and can sweep across the country and around the world in a very short time.

Wherever and whenever a pandemic starts, everyone around the world is at risk. Countries might, through measures such as border closures and travel restrictions, delay arrival of the virus, but cannot stop it.

Pandemics happen when a novel influenza virus emerges that can infect and be efficiently transmitted between humans. Animals are the most likely reservoir for these emerging viruses; swine and avian viruses have played a role in the last four influenza pandemics. Three of these pandemic-causing viruses remain in circulation and two are responsible for the majority of influenza cases that pass through each year.

Pandemics have occurred intermittently over centuries. The last three pandemics, in 1918, 1957, and 1968 killed approximately 40 million, 2 million, and 1 million people worldwide, respectively. Although the timing cannot be predicted, history and science suggest that we will face one or more pandemics in this century.

The most recent pandemic threats stem from an unprecedented outbreak of avian influenza and swine influenza in Asia, Europe, and Mexico. While traditional control measures have been attempted, the viruses are unlikely to be eradicated soon. A notable and worrisome feature of both viruses is their ability to infect a wide range of hosts, including birds, pigs, and humans.

Modern advances in travel increase the risk of a world-wide pandemic exponentially, in a way that did not exist for previous outbreaks. Historically, pandemics traveled from continent to continent through travel on ships, resulting in a six to eight month lag time before the entire globe was exposed. Today, worldwide exposure to an epidemic can happen in a matter of hours or days. For example, someone infected with swine flu contracted in Mexico can board a flight to Houston. The infected person exposes passengers on the flight, which results in those individuals exposing the passengers on their connecting flights. Through the course of a single day, it's possible for the virus to be carried to multiple continents.

Though the rate of international spread would likely have no direct effect on mortality, simultaneous outbreaks strain worldwide supplies of medicine, medical supplies, and treatment, making it more difficult to contain the disease and effectively treat those affected. Additionally, increases in urban population densities worldwide mean that more people will be exposed to the virus during everyday activities than during previous pandemics.

Once a flu pandemic takes hold, under current technologies, it will take several months before a vaccine to the specific virus will be widely available. After receiving a vaccine, in can take two to six weeks for the inoculation to work against the virus.

A New Outbreak

If a worldwide epidemic does not occur with the current circulating strain of flu viruses, history suggests that a different influenza virus will emerge that will.

Preparing for a pandemic requires the leveraging of all instruments of national power, and coordinated action by all segments of government and society. Influenza viruses do not respect the distinctions of race, sex, age, profession, or nationality, and are not constrained by geographic boundaries. The next pandemic is likely to come in waves, each lasting months, and pass through communities of all size across the nation and world. While a pandemic will not damage power lines, banks, or computer networks, it will ultimately threaten all critical infrastructures by removing essential personnel from the workplace for weeks or months.

This makes a pandemic a unique circumstance necessitating a strategy that extends well beyond health and medical boundaries to include: the sustainment of critical infrastructure, private-sector activities, the movement of goods and services across the nation and the globe, and economic and security considerations. The uncertainties associated with influenza viruses require that any strategy be versatile, to ensure that we are prepared for any virus with pandemic potential, as well as the annual burden of influenza that we know we will face.

Economic Impacts of a Global Flu Pandemic

A worldwide flu pandemic could have a major effect on the global economy including travel, trade, tourism, food, consumption, and eventually, investment and financial markets. The potential economic impacts presented below are based on a report from the Congressional Budget Office.

Short-Term Effects
The most immediate impact of a pandemic would be a surge in demand for medical services. During a severe pandemic, hospitals, clinics, and doctors' offices will be overwhelmed, and surveillance (keeping track of where the disease is and where it was going) will be difficult. Health care workers will be exposed to the disease, resulting in further strains on the health care system, as some workers become sick and others stay home to care for family members or to avoid becoming ill.

Care for less immediate health problems will be sharply curtailed. As the pandemic progresses, international travel will

Global Time Bomb

dramatically decline, as people avoid flu "hotspots" and governments restrict travel. It seems unlikely that domestic and international air travel will cease completely, but as a point of reference, at the peak of the SARS outbreak in April 2003, airline passenger arrivals in Hong Kong declined by nearly two-thirds.

In all likelihood, people will quarantine themselves and their families by staying at home. Nonessential activities that require social contact will be sharply cut, which will lead to significant declines in retail and restaurant sales. People will avoid public places such as shopping malls, community centers, places of worship, and public transit. Attendance at theaters, sporting events, museums, and restaurants will decline. It is likely that many schools will close, and if they do not, attendance will fall dramatically as parents keep their children at home. In either event, large-scale school closings will lead to a spike in workplace absences because even parents who are not sick will stay home to care for their children who are.

The general slowdown in economic activity will reduce gross domestic product (GDP). Business confidence will be dented; the supply of labor will be restricted (owing to illness, mortality, and absenteeism spurred by fear of contracting the disease); supply chains will be strained as transportation systems are disrupted; late payments and default rates on consumer and business debt will likely rise. It seems quite likely that the stock market will fall initially and then rebound later, as it did in Hong Kong during the SARS episode. Of course, economic activity will slow, but it will not halt completely.

Experience with such catastrophes as natural disasters and terrorist attacks has demonstrated the ability of people to cope with and adapt to extremely difficult circumstances. Moreover, the advances in technology of recent years will allow many companies, especially those in service industries, to conduct business via electronic communications, which will permit employees to work from home. And to the degree that shipping companies are operating, on-line purchases may offset some of the decline in retail trade.

The actions of governments could influence the effects of a pandemic on the economy. Attempts to quarantine people will probably amplify the reductions in trade, travel, and tourism. However, government actions may also help mitigate economic impacts. Effective global surveillance and prompt identification of the pandemic strain by government agencies—along with quarantine and social isolation—may provide the opportunity for manufacturers to develop a vaccine to lessen the human and economic costs of the pandemic during its latter stages.

Long-Term Effects

The most important long-term impact of a pandemic would be the reduction in the population and in the labor force after overall demand in the economy returned to normal. The effects of that drop in population would depend, in part, on the characteristics of the outbreak. If, for example, mortality was concentrated among the very young and the very old, then a pandemic would have relatively small effects on the subsequent growth of the economy. By contrast, if the disease struck people in their prime working years, the effects on economic growth during the years following the pandemic would be more significant. Under standard assumptions, a one-time reduction in the labor force would slow the pace of economic growth for many years.

Pandemic of 1918 (Spanish Flu)

In 1890, an especially virulent influenza pandemic struck, killing many Americans. Those who survived that pandemic and lived to experience the 1918 pandemic tended to be less susceptible to the disease. The pandemic which occurred in 1918-1919 was not the only influenza pandemic of the twentieth century. Influenza returned in a pandemic form in 1957-1958 and, again, in 1968-1969.

By May of 1918, reports of severe influenza trickled in from Europe. Within two months, influenza had spread from the military to the civilian population in Europe. From there, the disease spread outward—to Asia, Africa, South America and, back again, to North America. In late August, the influenza virus probably mutated again and epidemics erupted in three port cities: Freetown, Sierra Leone; Brest, France; and Boston, Massachusetts.

In Boston, dockworkers at Commonwealth Pier reported sick in massive numbers during the last week in August. Suffering from fevers as high as 105 degrees, these workers had severe muscle and joint pains. For most of these men, recovery quickly followed. But 5 to 10% of these patients developed severe and massive pneumonia. Death often followed.

Public health experts had little time to register their shock at the severity of this outbreak. Within days, the disease had spread outward to the city of Boston itself. By mid-September, the epidemic had spread even further with states as far away as California, North Dakota, Florida, and Texas reporting severe epidemics.

The pandemic of 1918-1919 occurred in three waves. The first wave had occurred when mild influenza erupted in the late spring and summer of 1918. The second wave occurred with an outbreak of severe influenza in the fall of 1918, and the final wave occurred in the spring of 1919. In its wake, the pandemic would leave about twenty million dead across the world. In America alone, about 675,000 people in a population of 105 million would die from the disease.

In Philadelphia, a city especially hard hit, so many children were orphaned that the Bureau of Child Hygiene found itself overwhelmed and unable to care for them. As the disease spread, schools and businesses emptied. Telegraph and telephone services collapsed as operators took to their beds. Garbage went uncollected as garbage men reported sick. The mail piled up as postal carriers failed to come to work.

State and local departments of health also suffered from high absentee rates. No one was left to record the pandemic's spread and the Public Health Service's requests for information went unanswered. As the bodies accumulated, funeral parlors ran out of caskets and bodies went uncollected in morgues. In the absence of a sure cure, fighting influenza seemed an impossible task.

In many communities, quarantines were imposed to prevent the spread of the disease. Schools, theaters, saloons, pool halls, and even churches were closed. As the bodies mounted, even funerals were held outdoors to protect mourners against the spread of the disease.

In November, two months after the pandemic had erupted, the Public Health Service began reporting that influenza cases were declining. Communities slowly lifted their quarantines. Masks were discarded. Schools were re-opened and citizens flocked to celebrate the end of World War I. Communities and the disease continued to be a threat throughout the spring of 1919.

Effects of the Pandemic

By the time the pandemic ended in the summer of 1919, nearly 675,000 Americans were dead from influenza. Hundreds of thousands more were orphaned and widowed.

During the 1920s, researchers estimated that 21.5 million people died as a result of the 1918-1919 pandemic. More recent estimates show global mortality from the 1918-1919 pandemic at anywhere between 30 and 50 million. An estimated 675,000 Americans were among the dead. All of these deaths caused a severe disruption in the economy. Claims against life insurance policies skyrocketed, with one insurance company reporting a 745 percent rise in the number of claims made. Small businesses, many of which had been unable to operate during the pandemic, went bankrupt.

In the summer and fall of 1919, Americans called for the government to research both the causes and impact of the pandemic. In response, both the federal government and private companies, such as Metropolitan Life Insurance, dedicated money specifically for flu research. In an attempt to determine the effect influenza had in different communities, the Public Health Service conducted several small epidemiological studies. These studies, however, were conducted after the pandemic and most PHS officers admitted that the data collected was probably inaccurate.

PHS scientists continued to search for the causative agent of influenza in their laboratories, as did their fellow scientists in and outside the United States. But while there was a burst of enthusiasm for funding flu research in 1918-1919, the funds allocated for this research were actually fairly meager. As time passed, Americans became less interested in the pandemic and its causes. And even when funding for medical research dramatically increased after World War II, funding for research on the 1918-1919 pandemic remained limited.

In the years following 1919, Americans seemed eager to forget the pandemic. Given the devastating impact of the pandemic, the reasons for this forgetfulness are puzzling. It is possible, however, that the pandemic's close association with World War I may have caused this amnesia. While more people died from the pandemic than from World War I, the war had lasted longer than the pandemic and caused greater and more immediate changes in American society.

Influenza also hit communities quickly. Often it disappeared within a few weeks of its arrival. As one historian put it, "the disease moved fast, arrived, flourished and was gone before many people had time to fully realize just how great was the danger." Small wonder, then, that many Americans forgot about the pandemic in the years that followed.

The Search for Understanding

In the early stages of the pandemic, many scientists believed that the agent responsible for influenza was Pfeiffer's bacillus. Autopsies and research conducted during the pandemic ultimately led many scientists to discard this theory.

In 1918, most physicians and scientists mistakenly believed that influenza was caused by a bacteria, not a virus. Called *Pfeiffer's bacillus*, this bacteria had been first identified as the cause of influenza by Robert Friedrich Pfeiffer, a leading German scientist. Although Pfeiffer had failed to provide definitive proof that this bacillus actually caused influenza, few scientists questioned his claims. In the midst of the pandemic, however, this theory came under attack. Researchers performing autopsies on influenza victims reported, over and over again, that they had failed to locate the bacteria. Attempts to infect healthy patients with influenza by injecting them with Pfeiffer's bacillus also failed to cause influenza.

Although they were unable to locate the cause of influenza, scientists and physicians did understand that influenza was spread through contact with droplets from the nose and throat of an infected person during coughing and sneezing. Most early twentieth-century physicians were familiar with influenza and its symptoms. Diagnosis, however, was often difficult as physicians frequently confused the disease with another viral infection, the common cold. In 1918, diagnosing influenza became even more difficult because an especially virulent form of the disease had erupted.

Early symptoms of the disease now included a temperature in the range of 102 to 104 degrees. Along with this high temperature, patients also experienced a sore throat, exhaustion, headache, aching limbs, bloodshot eyes, a cough, and occasionally a violent nosebleed. Some patients also suffered from digestive symptoms such as vomiting or diarrhea. Most patients who experienced these symptoms made a full recovery. Many patients recovered only to suffer a relapse. Their temperatures, which had fallen, rose again and they now experienced serious respiratory problems. In some cases, these patients also experienced massive pulmonary hemorrhages. After death, pathologists found these victims to have swollen lungs and oversized spleens.

Because patients experienced symptoms not traditionally associated with influenza, physicians found the disease especially difficult to diagnose in 1918. In the early stages of the pandemic, many physicians and scientists even claimed that influenza patients were suffering from cholera or bubonic plague, not influenza. Before the advent of antibiotics in the 1940s, practitioners had only a limited ability to treat diseases. Moreover, even if antibiotics had been available in 1918, a viral disease such as influenza could not have been treated by these drugs.

In late October of 1918, some researchers began to argue that influenza was caused by a virus. Although scientists had understood that viruses could cause diseases for more than two decades, virology was still very much in its infancy at this time. It was not until 1933 that the influenza A virus, which causes almost every type of endemic and pandemic influenza, was isolated. Seven years later, in 1940, the influenza B virus was isolated. The influenza C virus was finally isolated in 1950.

Influenza vaccine was first introduced as a licensed product in the United States in 1944. Because of the rapid rate of mutation of the influenza virus, the effectiveness of a given vaccine usually lasts for only a year or two. By the 1950s, vaccine makers were able to prepare and routinely release vaccines which could be used in the prevention or control of future pandemics. During the 1960s, increased understanding of the virus enabled scientists to develop both more potent and purer vaccines. Mass production of influenza vaccines continued, however, to require several months lead time.

During the mid to late nineteenth-century, physicians and scientists had begun to understand that microorganisms cause diseases. This was a radical departure from traditional medical theories which had held that diseases were caused by miasmas or an imbalance in the body's humors. Building on this new understanding of disease, scientists and physicians achieved incredible successes, identifying fifty causative agents of diseases ranging from typhoid, tuberculosis, cholera, plague, and malaria between 1880 and 1920.

2

Managing Flu Viruses

Humans can be infected with influenza types A, B, and C viruses. Subtypes of influenza A that are currently circulating among people worldwide include H1N1, H1N2, and H3N2 viruses.

Wild birds are the natural host for all known subtypes of influenza A viruses. Typically, wild birds do not become sick when they are infected with avian influenza A viruses. However, domestic poultry, such as turkeys and chickens, can become very sick and die from avian flu.

Low versus Highly Pathogenic Avian Influenza A Viruses
Avian influenza A virus strains are further classified as low pathogenic (LPAI) or highly pathogenic (HPAI) on the basis of specific molecular genetic and pathogenesis criteria that require specific testing. Most avian influenza A viruses are LPAI viruses that are usually associated with mild disease in poultry. In

contrast, HPAI viruses can cause severe illness and high mortality in poultry.

In general, human infection with avian influenza viruses has been associated with direct contact with infected live or dead birds (domestic poultry).

How Flu Viruses Change

Influenza viruses are dynamic and are continuously evolving. They can change in two different ways: antigenic drift and antigenic shift. Influenza viruses are changing by antigenic drift all the time, but antigenic shift happens only occasionally. Type A viruses undergo both kinds of changes; type B viruses change only by the more gradual process of antigenic drift.

Antigenic drift refers to small, gradual changes that occur through mutations. These mutations occur unpredictably and result in minor changes to the virus. Antigenic drift produces new virus strains that may not be recognized by antibodies to earlier influenza strains. This process works as follows: a person infected with a particular flu strain develops antibody against that strain. As newer strains appear, the antibodies against the older strains might not recognize the "newer" virus, and infection with a new strain can occur. This is one of the main reasons why people can become infected with influenza viruses more than one time. In most years, one or two of the three virus strains in the influenza vaccine are updated to keep up with the changes in the circulating flu viruses. For this reason, people who want to be immunized against influenza need to be vaccinated every year.

Antigenic shift refers to an abrupt, major change to produce a novel flu virus in humans not currently circulating among people. Antigenic shift can occur either through direct animal-to-human transmission or through mixing of human influenza A and animal influenza A virus genes to create a new human flu virus through a process called genetic reassortment. This is what appears to have occurred with the swine flu H1N1 virus of 2009. Antigenic shift results in a new human influenza. A global influenza pandemic (worldwide spread) may occur if three conditions are met:

- A new flu virus is introduced into the human population.
- The virus causes serious illness in humans.
- The virus can spread easily from person to person in a sustained manner.

Influenza Pandemic Preparedness

The biggest concern and most serious health threat over the flu is the possibility of it becoming a global pandemic that could be difficult or impossible to control.

The H5N1 bird flu virus that emerged in Asia and Europe meets the first two conditions: it is a new virus for humans (H5N1 viruses have never circulated widely among people), and it has infected more than 190 humans, killing over half of them.

However, the third condition, the establishment of efficient and sustained human-to-human transmission of the virus, has not occurred. For this to take place, the H5N1 virus would need to improve its transmissibility among humans. This could occur either by reassortment or adaptive mutation.

Reassortment occurs when genetic material is exchanged between human and avian viruses during co-infection (infection with both viruses at the same time) of a human or another mammal. The result could be a fully transmissible pandemic virus—that is, a virus that can spread easily and directly between humans. A more gradual process is adaptive mutation, where the capability of a virus to bind to human cells increases during infections of humans.

The H1N1 swine flu is thought to be the result of reassortment of genetic material between three influenza viruses: the bird flu, swine flu, and human flu. Because this flu meets the three requirements named above, the conditions for a serious global flu pandemic have been met.

To prepare for such a pandemic, the Centers for Disease Control has already taken part in a number of pandemic prevention and preparedness activities. Because of the 2005 avian flu scare, the CDC began aggressive efforts to deal with what soon became a pandemic.

The CDC is working closely with the World Health Organization (WHO) and the National Institutes of Health on safety testing of vaccine candidates and development of additional vaccine virus seed candidates for other types of influenza A viruses.

Isolation and Quarantine

To contain the spread of a contagious illness, public health authorities rely on many strategies. Two of these strategies are isolation and quarantine. Both are common practices in public health, and both aim to control exposure to infected or potentially infected persons. Both may be undertaken voluntarily or compelled by public health authorities. The two strategies differ in that isolation applies to persons who are known to have an illness, and quarantine applies to those who have been exposed to an illness but who may or may not become ill.

During the 2003 global SARS outbreak, for example, patients in the United States were isolated until they were no longer infectious. This practice allowed patients to receive appropriate care, and it helped contain the spread of the illness. Seriously ill patients were cared for in hospitals. Persons with mild illness were cared for at home. Persons being cared for at home were asked to avoid contact with other people and to remain at home until ten days after the resolution of fever, provided respiratory symptoms were absent or improving.

In the United States, where there was limited transmission of SARS, neither individual nor population-based quarantine of contacts was recommended. The CDC advised persons who were exposed but not symptomatic to monitor themselves for symptoms and advised home isolation and medical evaluation if symptoms appeared. Individual quarantine was an integral part of the control measures used in countries more severely affected by the outbreak. Quarantine of large groups was used only in selected settings where extensive transmission was occurring.

Thanks to these efforts and others, a mere eight months after the disease broke out, new cases became non-existent and the WHO was able to declare the global outbreak to be over.

Isolation for people who are ill

Isolation refers to the separation of persons who have a specific infectious illness from those who are healthy and the restriction of their movement to stop the spread of that illness. Isolation allows for the focused delivery of specialized health care to people who are ill, and it protects healthy people from getting sick. People in isolation may be cared for in their homes, in hospitals, or in designated healthcare facilities. Isolation is a standard procedure used in hospitals today for patients with tuberculosis (TB) and certain other infectious diseases. In most cases, isolation is voluntary; however, many levels of government (federal, state, and local) have basic authority to compel isolation of sick people to protect the public.

Quarantine for people who have been exposed but are not ill

Quarantine refers to the separation and restriction of movement of persons who, while not yet ill, have been exposed to an infectious agent and therefore may become infectious. Quarantine of exposed persons is a public health strategy, like isolation, quarantine is intended to stop the spread of infectious disease. Quarantine is medically very effective in protecting the public from disease.

States generally have authority to declare and enforce quarantine within their borders. This authority varies widely from state to state, depending on state laws. The CDC, through its Division of Global Migration and Quarantine, also is empowered to detain, medically examine, or conditionally release persons suspected of carrying certain communicable diseases. This authority derives from section 361 of the Public Health Service Act (42 U.S.C. 264), as amended.

3

H3N2v (Swine Flu)

NOTICE: *The information given in this chapter is based on the most readily available information at the time of publishing. Because this is a relatively new disease, some of the information given may change or become outdated. Check www.CDC.gov for the most current information.*

H3N2v Background

In the second half of 2011, a number of U.S. residents were found to be infected with influenza A variant viruses, primarily H3N2v. Investigations revealed human infections with these viruses following contact with swine as well as limited human-to-human transmission. These viruses are substantially different from human influenza A (H3N2) viruses, so the seasonal vaccine is expected to provide limited cross-protection among adults and no protection to children.

While H3N2v viruses have been detected in U.S. swine, it's unknown how widespread they are in swine herds. It's possible that sporadic infections and even localized outbreaks among people with this virus will continue to occur. So far, the severity of illnesses associated with this virus in people has been similar to the severity of illnesses associated with seasonal flu virus infections. Limited serologic studies indicate that adults may have some pre-existing immunity to this virus while children do not.

Variant Influenza Viruses

Swine flu viruses do not normally infect humans. However, sporadic human infections with influenza viruses that normally circulate in swine and not people have occurred. When this happens, these viruses are called "variant viruses." They also can be denoted by adding the letter "v" to the end of the virus subtype designation. Human infections with H1N1v, H3N2v and H1N2v viruses have been detected in the United States.

Most commonly, human infections with variant viruses occur in people with exposure to infected pigs (e.g. children near pigs at a fair or workers in the swine industry). There have been documented cases of multiple persons becoming sick after exposure to one or more sick pigs and also cases of limited spread of variant influenza viruses from person-to-person. The vast majority of human infections with variant influenza viruses do not result in person-to-person spread. However, each case of human infection with a swine influenza virus should be fully investigated to be sure that such viruses are not spreading in an efficient and ongoing way in humans and to limit further exposure of humans to infected animals if infected animals are identified.

Editorial Note

Human infections with the influenza viruses currently circulating among swine are rare. Since 2005, only 35 cases have been reported in the United States, but the frequency with which they have been detected increased in 2011. When different influenza viruses simultaneously infect a single host (e.g., a human or swine), exchange of genetic material can occur, resulting in a new influenza virus. Depending on the antigenic distance between the new virus and recently circulating seasonal viruses, little or no immunity might exist in the human population. Influenza A (H3N2)v viruses resulted from reassortment of influenza A (H1N1)pdm09 viruses with swine influenza A (H3N2) viruses. A diagram depicting this reassortment is available online from CDC's Public Health Image Library.§ Because these viruses carry a newly identified combination of genes, little information is available regarding transmission efficiency in swine, in humans, or between swine and humans. However, the recent human cases involving swine exposure and results of SIV surveillance indicate that these viruses also currently are circulating in swine herds.

The case of influenza A (H3N2)v infection after occupational contact with swine in Indiana and the apparent limited human-to-human transmission of A(H3N2)v virus that occurred in a day care setting in West Virginia represent two different possible scenarios for transmission of this virus. Work exposure highlights the risk for interspecies influenza transmission in occupational settings where humans are exposed to swine, an association that has been described previously (3–7). To minimize the risk for interspecies influenza transmission in occupational settings, CDC and the Occupational Safety and Health Administration (OSHA) encourage swine workers to 1) get vaccinated against human seasonal influenza, 2) wear appropriate PPE, and 3) practice good hygiene, such as washing hands thoroughly with soap and water, when in contact with swine, especially swine that show signs of illness. The National Pork Board also recommends producers work with their veterinarian to develop appropriate prevention and control measures for influenza in swine, which can include vaccinating swine against swine influenza. Similar to humans, swine infected with influenza viruses do not always exhibit signs of infection (8). Persons with swine exposure in the week before onset of an illness with symptoms of influenza requiring medical care should notify their health-care provider of their swine exposures. Persons who develop symptoms of influenza after close contact with swine are recommended to stay home until well to minimize contact with persons and swine as much as possible.

The A(H3N2)v cases in West Virginia involved two children who attended the same day care, but the first child was unlikely to have transmitted the virus to the second child, given the ≥10-day difference in their symptom onset dates. This represents a scenario of limited human-to-human transmission occurring in a day care setting. Therefore, clinicians also should consider the possibility of influenza A (H3N2)v infections in patients who have not had exposure to swine, particularly young children in those states where influenza A (H3N2)v cases have been reported. Clinicians who suspect variant influenza virus infection should obtain a nasopharyngeal swab, place the swab in viral transport medium, and contact their state or local health department to facilitate transport and timely diagnosis. Influenza A (H3N2)v viruses detected to date are susceptible to oseltamivir and zanamivir for the treatment of influenza. Clinicians who suspect variant influenza infection in a patient should consider treatment with these medications if clinically indicated. Because these viruses have the M gene from the influenza A (H1N1)pdm09 virus, they are resistant to amantadine and rimantadine. CDC requests that state public health laboratories notify CDC immediately of suspected variant influenza A specimens and send them to the CDC Influenza Division's Virus Surveillance and Diagnostics Branch Laboratory. Confirmed cases should be investigated thoroughly and expeditiously to ascertain whether swine-to-human or human-to-human transmission is ongoing and to limit further exposures between humans with others and swine. Such investigations require close collaboration among state, local, and federal public and animal health officials.

CDC is working with USDA and state public health and animal health experts in the locations where these cases have occurred to investigate each case fully and to enhance influenza surveillance to detect human cases of variant influenza virus infections. The CDC rRT-PCR assay that was approved by the Food and Drug Administration in September 2011 is able to identify these cases as presumptive influenza A (H3N2)v cases. These diagnostic test kits have been distributed to public health laboratories in the United States and National Influenza Centers designated by the World Health Organization in other countries. Additional rRT-PCR test enhancements to further improve detection of influenza A (H3N2)v viruses are under development.

Limited serologic studies conducted to date indicate that young children have little preexisting immunity to influenza A (H3N2)v viruses. Because the hemagglutinin genes of these viruses are related to human influenza A (H3N2) viruses that circulated in the 1990s, older children and adults might have limited immunity against these viruses. Certain persons, including young children, pregnant women, persons with chronic health conditions such as asthma, diabetes, or heart and lung disease, and persons aged ≥65 years, are likely to be at greater risk for serious influenza-related complications from variant influenza viruses such as influenza A (H3N2)v. The influenza A (H3N2)v virus is different enough from current human seasonal influenza viruses that the seasonal influenza vaccine is not expected to provide significant protection.

Prevention Strategies for H3N2v in Health Care Settings

Influenza A(H3N2)variant [A(H3N2)v] virus is an influenza virus that contains genes from human, avian and swine origins. As of 23 December, 2011, the virus has been detected in 12 persons in the U.S., all since July 2011. Most infections with this virus have resulted in self-limited, mild respiratory illnesses; however, three persons have been hospitalized. None have died. While it is unknown whether this virus will continue to occur among humans or become more common, it is possible that health care providers will care for patients that are infected with this virus. There are no data to indicate that the transmission characteristics of the A(H3N2)v virus will be different than those of seasonal influenza viruses. As a result, CDC advises that the infections control principles and actions relevant for seasonal influenza are appropriate for the control of A(H3N2)v as well.

Of special note is that the current infection control guidance recommends vaccination of health care workers and patients as a critical step to reduce seasonal influenza transmission in these settings. Current CDC data indicate that seasonal vaccines may provide limited protection against infection with A(H3N2)v viruses among adults and no protection in children. While the effectiveness of current seasonal vaccines to protect against A(H3N2)v virus infections might be reduced compared with effectiveness of seasonal vaccines against seasonal influenza, CDC recommends their use. They remain the best tool for the prevention of seasonal influenza transmission in health care settings, which is currently the greatest risk from influenza during this influenza season.

Surveillance

In recent weeks, human infections with an influenza A(H3N2) variant ([H3N2]v)virus have been identified in 5 states: West Virginia, Indiana, Pennsylvania, Maine, and Iowa. The epidemiology of some of the identified clusters is suggestive of limited person-to-person transmission. Documented illnesses have occurred mostly in children, leading to the concern that children, primarily those in elementary school and younger, may have increased susceptibility to these influenza viruses.

This section provides interim guidance for state and local health departments, hospitals, and clinicians participating in surveillance activities regarding patients targeted for enhanced surveillance and testing by real-time reverse transcriptase-polymerase chain reaction (rRT-PCR) for influenza. Use of rRT-PCR testing is important for surveillance in order to identify which influenza A subtypes (e.g. influenza A(H3N2)v versus seasonal H1N1 or H3N2 viruses) are circulating. Due to the ongoing identification of patients with influenza A(H3N2)v virus infection this fall, these guidelines have been developed in an effort to facilitate timely detection and investigation of cases by targeting patients for influenza testing by rRT-PCR for surveillance.

CDC would like state and local health departments to consider the following recommendations for influenza surveillance and testing.

1. All public health laboratories should use the CDC Human Influenza Real-Time rRT-PCR Diagnostic Panel to screen specimens for InfA, InfB, and RP. Then test all InfA-positive specimens with the CDC Influenza A Subtyping kit

using all primer/probe sets: H1, H3, pdmInfA and pdmH1. Detailed guidance for testing can be found in the influenza surveillance diagnostic testing algorithm disseminated recently by APHL.

2. Contact tracing of confirmed, probable, or suspected influenza A(H3N2)v cases should be completed to gather more information about the epidemiology of the virus and modes of transmission.

3. Currently, while there are low levels of circulating seasonal influenza viruses, CDC recommends increasing collection of specimens from patients with influenza-like illness (ILI) , and having these specimens sent to the state or local laboratory for prioritization for rRT-PCR testing. States should specifically consider increasing collection of specimens from patients presenting with ILI in the following high priority areas:

    a. ILI outbreaks, particularly among children in child-care and school settings, since these have been the settings associated with human-to-human influenza A(H3N2)v virus transmission.

    b. Unusual or severe presentations of ILI, especially among children.

    c. Medically attended ILI and ARI in children under 18 years of age

Specimen Collection, Processing, and Testing for Suspect H3N2

- Case Definitions
- Duration of Viral Shedding
- Testing for Influenza A (H3N2)v Virus
- Preferred Respiratory Specimens
- Swabs
- Storing Clinical Specimens

- Shipping Clinical Specimens
- Diagnostic Testing

This section is intended for public health professionals to provide interim guidance on appropriate specimen collection, storage, processing, and testing for patients with suspected influenza A (H3N2) variant ([H3N2]v) virus infection. These guidelines for specimen collection, storage, processing, and shipping are consistent with guidance for the submission of seasonal influenza viruses to the laboratory.

Duration of Viral Shedding
The duration of shedding of influenza A (H3N2)v virus is unknown. Therefore, until data are available, the estimated duration of viral shedding is based upon seasonal influenza virus infection. Infected persons should be assumed to be contagious up to 7 days from illness onset. Infected persons can shed virus and are potentially infectious from the day prior to illness onset until resolution of fever. Some persons who are infected might shed virus and be contagious for longer periods (e.g. young infants and immunocompromised persons).

Testing for Influenza A (H3N2)v Virus
Clinicians should consider testing suspected cases of influenza A (H3N2)v virus infection, especially those with severe illness, by obtaining an upper respiratory specimen.

Preferred Respiratory Specimens
The following should be collected as soon as possible after illness onset: nasopharyngeal swab, nasal aspirate or wash or a combined nasopharyngeal swab with oropharyngeal swab. If these specimens cannot be collected, a nasal swab or oropharyngeal swab is acceptable. For patients who are intubated, an endotracheal aspirate should also be collected. Bronchoalveolar

lavage (BAL) and sputum specimens are also acceptable. Specimens should be placed into sterile viral transport media and immediately placed on refrigerant gel-packs or at 4°C (refrigerator) for transport to the laboratory.

Swabs

Ideally, swab specimens should be collected using swabs with a synthetic tip (e.g., polyester or Dacron®) and an aluminum or plastic shaft. Swabs with cotton tips and wooden shafts are not recommended. Specimens collected with swabs made of calcium alginate are not acceptable. The swab specimen collection vials should contain 1-3ml of viral transport medium (e.g., containing, protein stabilizer, antibiotics to discourage bacterial and fungal growth, and buffer solution).

Storing Clinical Specimens

Respiratory specimens should be kept at 4°C for no longer than 3 days. Specimens can alternatively be frozen at ≤-70°C. Avoid freezing and thawing specimens if at all possible.

Shipping Clinical Specimens

Clinical specimens should be shipped to the laboratory in the appropriate packaging. If clinical specimens will be examined within 72 hours after collection, keep the specimen at 4°C (2-8 °C) and ship on refrigerant gel-packs, otherwise store frozen at ≤-70°C and ship on dry ice. Avoid freezing and thawing specimens. Viability of some pathogens from specimens that were frozen and then thawed is greatly diminished.

All specimens should be labeled clearly and include information requested by your state public health laboratory. Suspected influenza A (H3N2)v specimens shipped from the state public health laboratory to CDC should include all information required for seasonal influenza surveillance isolate or specimen submission.

Diagnostic Testing

The performance of current Food and Drug Administration (FDA) cleared diagnostic tests for influenza has been demonstrated for seasonal human influenza viruses as described by the manufacturer package insert. Performance has not been demonstrated with novel influenza A viruses; these viruses only infect humans sporadically. However, some diagnostic assays may detect the presence of novel influenza A viruses.

Molecular assays may detect novel influenza A viruses, but will not differentiate novel influenza A viruses from seasonal influenza A viruses. For these assays a novel influenza A virus:

- May give an influenza A "unsubtypable" result. Clinicians and laboratorians using molecular assays that are capable of detecting all currently circulating influenza A subtypes who identify an "unsubtypable" result should contact their state or local public health laboratory for additional testing.
- May give a false positive result for human influenza A(H3) viruses

Rapid influenza diagnostic tests (RIDTs) and immunofluorescence tests also have unknown sensitivity and specificity to detect human infection with influenza A (H3N2)v virus in clinical specimens. These tests may give a positive influenza A result for a specimen containing influenza A (H3N2)v virus. However, negative results from either type of test do not exclude influenza virus infection in patients with signs and symptoms suggestive of influenza. Therefore, a negative test result could be a false negative and should not be assumed a final diagnostic test for influenza A (H3N2)v virus infection.

Specimens from suspected influenza A (H3N2)v cases should be evaluated first by qualified public health laboratories prior to sending to CDC, if possible. Influenza A (H3N2)v viruses will be positive for the nucleoprotein (NP) gene target (pdmInfA) of the CDC Human Influenza Real-Time RT-PCR Diagnostic Panel as well as for the influenza A and seasonal influenza A (H3) targets. Qualified public health laboratories obtaining this result should contact the CDC, Influenza Division, Virus Surveillance and Diagnostic Branch Laboratory immediately. All suspected novel influenza A viruses and influenza A (H3N2)v specimens should be sent to CDC for confirmatory testing. Confirmation of influenza A (H3N2)v virus is performed only at CDC at this time.

Note: Antiviral treatment should not be withheld from patients with suspected influenza if the patient is hospitalized, has severe or progressive illness, or the patient has an underlying condition that places them at increased risk for influenza-related complications, even if they test negative for influenza.

Investigations of Influenza A(H3N2)v Cases

This section provides updated interim guidance for state and local health departments conducting investigations of infections with influenza A (H3N2) variant [(H3N2)v] viruses. The following case definitions are for the purpose of investigations of suspected, probable, and confirmed cases of influenza A (H3N2)v virus infection. CDC is requesting notification of all suspected and probable cases of influenza A (H3N2)v virus infection within 24 hours of identification. When possible, state health departments are encouraged to investigate suspected cases of influenza A (H3N2)v virus infection further to determine case status.

Case Definitions for Infection with Influenza A (H3N2)v Virus

A *suspected case* of influenza A (H3N2)v virus infection is defined as acute respiratory illness (ARI) in a person who:

- Is epidemiologically linked to a confirmed case of influenza A (H3N2)v virus infection (see below).

OR

- Has had illness onset within 7 days of swine exposure.

Acute respiratory illness (ARI) is defined as recent onset of at least **two** of the following:

- Rhinorrhea or nasal congestion
- Sore throat
- Cough
- Fever or feverishness

A *probable case* of influenza A (H3N2)v virus infection is defined as ARI in a person who:

- Had a specimen tested using the CDC Human Influenza Virus real-time reverse-transcriptase polymerase chain reaction (rRT-PCR) Diagnostic Panel and is **positive** for InfA, pdmInfA, and H3; and **negative** for InfB, pdmH1, and H1.

OR

- Is epidemiologically linked to a confirmed case of influenza A (H3N2)v, and for whom results of influenza diagnostic testing of an appropriate respiratory specimen are **positive** for influenza A (H3) or **positive** for influenza A (no subtype tested or detected).

A **confirmed case** of influenza A (H3N2)v virus infection is defined as influenza A (H3N2)v virus infection in a person that is laboratory-confirmed at CDC.

Guidance for School Administrators

- Background
- High-Risk Groups
- Symptoms and Emergency Warning Signs
- Recommendations
- Additional Resources

This section, based on recommendations from the Centers for Disease Control and Prevention (CDC), provides guidance to help reduce the spread of seasonal influenza (flu) among students and staff in K-12 schools. Recommendations are based on CDC's current knowledge of flu in the United States. CDC will continue to monitor flu activity and update this guidance as needed.

For the purpose of this guidance, "schools" will refer to both public and private institutions providing grades K-12 education to children and adolescents in group settings.

Background

Flu seasons are unpredictable in a number of ways. Although widespread influenza activity occurs every year, the timing, severity, and duration of it depend on many factors, including which flu viruses are spreading, the number of people who are susceptible to the circulating flu viruses, and how well the flu vaccine is matched to the flu viruses that are causing illness. The timing of flu can vary from season to season. In the United States, seasonal flu activity most commonly peaks in January or February, but flu viruses can cause illness from early October to late May. Flu viruses are thought to spread mainly from person to person through coughs and sneezes of infected individuals. People may also become infected by touching something with flu virus on it and then touching their mouth, nose, or eyes.

Many respiratory infections spread from person to person and cause symptoms similar to those of flu. Therefore, the nonpharmaceutical recommendations in this section might help reduce the spread of not only flu, but also respiratory syncytial virus (RSV), rhinovirus, and other viruses and bacteria that can cause illness.

Each day, about 55 million students and 7 million staff attend the more than 130,000 public and private schools in the United States. By implementing the recommendations in this section, schools can help protect one-fifth of the country's population from flu. Collaboration is essential; CDC, the U.S. Department of Education, state/local public health and education agencies, schools, staff, students, families, businesses, and communities should work together to reduce the spread of flu and other respiratory infections.

High-Risk Groups
People of all ages get sick with flu. School-aged children are the group with the highest rates of flu illness. Groups at highest risk for severe flu-related illness, including being hospitalized or dying from flu, include:
- Children younger than 5 years of age, but especially children younger than 2 years of age
- Adults 65 years of age and older
- Pregnant women
- American Indians/Alaskan Natives
- People younger than 19 years of age who are receiving long-term aspirin therapy
- People who have certain medical conditions, including:

o Asthma
o Other chronic lung diseases (such as chronic obstructive pulmonary disease [COPD] and cystic fibrosis)
o Neurological and neurodevelopmental conditions (including disorders of the brain, spinal cord, peripheral nerve, and muscle, such as cerebral palsy, epilepsy [seizure disorders], stroke, intellectual disability [mental retardation], moderate to severe developmental delay, muscular dystrophy, and spinal cord injury).
o Heart disease (such as congenital heart disease, congestive heart failure, and coronary artery disease)
o Blood disorders (such as sickle cell disease)
o Endocrine disorders (such as diabetes mellitus)
o Kidney disorders
o Liver disorders
o Metabolic disorders (such as inherited metabolic disorders and mitochondrial disorders)
o Weakened immune systems due to disease or medication (such as HIV/AIDS, cancer, and chronic use of steroids)
o Morbid obesity (body mass index [BMI] of 40 or greater)

Symptoms and Emergency Warning Signs
The symptoms of flu can include:
- Fever (although not everyone with flu has a fever)
- Cough
- Sore throat
- Runny or stuffy nose
- Body aches
- Headache

- Chills
- Tiredness
- Sometimes diarrhea and vomiting

Emergency warning signs that indicate a person should get medical care right away include:
- In children:
  - Fast breathing or trouble breathing
  - Bluish skin color
  - Not drinking enough fluids
  - Not waking up or not interacting
  - Being so irritable that the child does not want to be held
  - Flu-like symptoms that improve but then return with fever and worse cough
  - Fever with rash
- In addition to the signs above, get medical help right away for any infant who has any of these signs:
  - Being unable to eat
  - Has trouble breathing
  - Has no tears when crying
  - Has significantly fewer wet diapers than normal
- In adults:
  - Difficulty breathing or shortness of breath
  - Pain or pressure in the chest or abdomen
  - Sudden dizziness
  - Confusion
  - Severe or persistent vomiting
  - Flu-like symptoms that improve but then return with fever and worse cough

Recommendations

Below are recommendations to help reduce the spread of flu in schools.

- **Encourage students, parents, and staff to get a yearly flu vaccine.**
  - o Teach students, parents, and staff that the single best way to protect against the flu is to get vaccinated each year.
    - Seasonal flu vaccination is recommended for everyone 6 months of age and older unless they have a specific contraindication to flu vaccine.
    - The seasonal flu vaccine protects against three influenza viruses that research indicates will be most common during the upcoming season. The viruses in the vaccine change each year based on international surveillance and scientists' estimations about which types and strains of viruses will circulate in a given year.
    - There are two types of seasonal flu vaccines.
      - One type is the "flu shot" (sometimes called TIV for "trivalent inactivated influenza vaccine"), an inactivated vaccine containing killed virus that is given with a needle, usually in the arm. The flu shot is approved for use in people 6 months of age and older, including healthy people, pregnant women, and people with chronic medical conditions.
      - The second type is the nasal spray vaccine (sometimes called LAIV for "live attenuated influenza vaccine"), a vaccine made with live, weakened

flu viruses that do not cause flu. This vaccine is approved for use in people 2-49 years of age who are not pregnant and who do not have health problems.

- Flu vaccines have a very good safety record. Over the years, hundreds of millions of Americans have received seasonal flu vaccines. The most common side effects following flu vaccinations are mild, such as soreness, redness, tenderness, or swelling where the shot was given.
- Vaccination efforts can start as soon as vaccination becomes available (usually in September) and should continue as long as flu viruses are spreading and causing illness in the community (usually until May).

o Consider offering seasonal flu vaccination to students at school. School vaccination clinics, which are often led by local public health department staff in partnership with schools, are an option for vaccinating school-aged children against flu. Vaccination of other groups (e.g., staff, home-schooled students, students attending nearby schools, family members, and other community members) may also be considered. Contact your local public health department for more information.

o **Encourage students, parents, and staff to take everyday preventive actions to stop the spread of germs.**

o Encourage respiratory etiquette among students and staff through education and the provision of supplies.

- Teach students and staff to cover coughs and sneezes with a tissue or their arm. If they use a tissue, they should put the used tissue in a trash can and wash their hands.
- Provide adequate supplies within easy reach, including tissues and no-touch trash cans.

o Encourage hand hygiene among students and staff through education, scheduled time for handwashing, and the provision of supplies.

- Teach students and staff to wash hands often with soap and water for 20 seconds, dry hands with a paper towel, and use the paper towel to turn off the faucet. If soap and water are not available and hands are not visibly dirty, an alcohol-based hand sanitizer containing at least 60% alcohol may be used.
- Include handwashing time in student schedules.
- Provide adequate supplies, including clean and functional handwashing stations, soap, paper towels, and alcohol-based hand sanitizer.

o Encourage students and staff to keep their hands away from their nose, mouth, and eyes.

o Encourage routine surface cleaning through education, policy, and the provision of supplies.

- Routinely clean surfaces and objects that are touched often, such as desks, countertops, doorknobs, computer keyboards, hands-on learning items, faucet handles, and phones. Empty trash cans as needed.

- Use general cleaning products that you normally use. Always follow product label directions. Additional disinfection beyond routine cleaning is not recommended.
- Provide adequate supplies, such as general EPA-registered cleaning products, gloves, disinfecting wipes, and no-touch trash cans.
- Match your cleaning activities to the types of germs you want to remove or kill.
    - Flu viruses are relatively fragile, so standard practices, such as cleaning with soap and water, can help remove and kill them.
    - Most studies have shown that the flu virus can live and potentially infect a person for only 2 to 8 hours after being deposited on a surface. Therefore, special sanitizing processes beyond routine cleaning, including closing schools to clean every surface in the building, are not necessary or recommended to slow the spread of flu, even during a flu outbreak.
    - Some schools may include other cleaning and disinfecting practices in their standard procedures to address germs that are not removed or killed by soap and water alone.
- Encourage students and staff to stay home when sick through education and policy.
    - Teach students, parents, and staff the importance of staying home when sick until at least 24 hours

after they no longer have a fever (100 degrees Fahrenheit or 37.8 degrees Celsius, measured by mouth) or signs of a fever (chills, feeling very warm, flushed appearance, or sweating) without the use of fever-reducing medicine.

- Review school policies, and consider revising those that make it difficult for students and staff to stay home when sick or when caring for others who are sick.
    - Implement flexible sick leave policies for students and staff.
    - Avoid the use of perfect attendance awards.
    - Cross-train staff so that others can cover for co-workers who need to stay home.
- **Educate students, parents, and staff on what to do if someone gets sick**.
    - Teach students, parents, and staff the signs and symptoms of flu, emergency warning signs, and high-risk groups. See lists at the beginning of this section.
        - Those who get flu-like symptoms at school should go home and stay home until at least 24 hours after they no longer have a fever or signs of a fever without the

use of fever-reducing medicine. Those who have emergency warning signs should get immediate medical care.

- Those who get flu-like symptoms and are at high risk of severe flu illness should ask a healthcare provider if they should be examined.

- Separate sick students and staff from others until they can be picked up to go home. When feasible, identify a "sick room" through which others do not regularly pass. The sick room should be separated from areas used by well students for routine health activities, such as picking up medications. Sick room staff should be limited in number and should not be at high risk for severe illness if they get sick.

- Encourage students, parents, and staff to take antiviral drugs if their healthcare provider prescribes them.

  - Antiviral drugs, called Relenza® and Tamiflu®, are drugs that can be prescribed by healthcare providers to treat the flu. These drugs can reduce the number of days that a person is sick, but not everyone needs to be treated.

- Antiviral drugs work best when started within the first 2 days of illness, but they may also help reduce the risk of severe illness even if started 2 or more days after onset of illness for persons who are hospitalized.
- Although most people will recover from flu without treatment, antiviral drugs are recommended for people with influenza who have an illness requiring being in the hospital; have a progressive, severe, or complicated illness; or are at high risk of severe flu because of an underlying medical condition or their age.

- **Establish relationships with state and local health officials for ongoing communication.**
  - Follow your local flu situation through close communication with state and local health officials.
  - Update emergency plans so that they are in place before an outbreak occurs.

4

H1N1 (Swine Flu)

NOTICE: *The information given in this chapter is based on the most readily available information at the time of publishing. Because this is a relatively new disease, some of the information given may change or become outdated. Check www.CDC.gov for the most current information.*

On April 29, 2009, the World Health Organization warned the world that the first influenza pandemic since 1968 was imminent. Human infections with the newly identified H1N1 "swine flu" were first identified in April 2009 with cases in the United States and Mexico. The virus was originally referred to as swine flu because laboratory testing showed that many of the genes were similar to influenza viruses that normally occur in pigs. But further study has shown that this new virus is very different from what normally circulates in pigs. The H1N1 virus has two genes from flu viruses that normally circulate in pigs in Europe and Asia, as well as avian genes *and* human genes. Scientists call this a "quadruple reassortant" virus. Because it is a brand new virus, there is little natural human resistance to it.

Like all influenza viruses, swine flu viruses change constantly. Pigs can be infected by avian flu and human flu viruses as well as swine flu viruses. When flu viruses from different species infect pigs, the viruses can reassort (i.e. swap genes), and new viruses that are a mix of swine, human, and/or avian influenza viruses can emerge. Over the years, different variations of swine flu viruses have emerged. At this time, there are four main influenza type A virus subtypes that have been isolated in pigs: H1N1, H1N2, H3N2, and H3N1. However, most of the recently isolated influenza viruses from pigs have been H1N1 viruses.

Swine flu viruses are endemic among pig populations in the United States and something that the industry deals with routinely. Outbreaks among pigs normally occur in colder weather months (late fall and winter) and sometimes with the introduction of new pigs into susceptible herds. Studies have shown that the swine flu H1N1 is common throughout pig populations worldwide, with 25 percent of animals showing antibody evidence of infection.

Though there have been small swine flu outbreaks among humans in the past, the current flu pandemic is different because the virus is a different strain. The new strain spreads easily to humans and is passed efficiently from human to human.

In March 2009, Swine flu broke out in Mexico City, and within days, it spread from Mexico into the United States and then across the globe. The Centers for Disease Control (CDC), in collaboration with public health officials in California and Texas, immediately began investigating cases of febrile respiratory illness caused by swine influenza H1N1 viruses.

The viruses contain a unique combination of gene segments that have not been reported previously in the U.S. or elsewhere. The autumn of 2009 showed unprecedented levels of influenza activity throughout the country, all cases believed to be H1N1.

Swine Flu Outbreaks in History

In September 1988, a previously healthy 32-year-old pregnant woman was hospitalized for pneumonia and died eight days later. A swine H1N1 flu virus was detected. Four days before getting sick, the patient visited a county fair swine exhibition where there was widespread influenza-like illness among the swine.

In follow-up studies, 76% of swine exhibitors tested had antibody evidence of swine flu infection but showed no signs of serious illnesses. Therefore, it is possible to be exposed to the virus without actually getting sick. Additional studies suggest that one to three health care personnel, who had contact with the patient, developed mild influenza-like illnesses with antibody evidence of swine flu infection.

Seriousness of the Disease

Like seasonal flu, swine flu in humans can vary in severity from mild to severe, and at times can lead to death. Each year in the United States, an average of 36,000 people die from seasonal flu-related complications and more than 200,000 people are hospitalized for flu-related causes. Of those hospitalized, 20,000 are children younger than five years old. Over 90 percent of deaths and about 60 percent of hospitalization occur in people older than 65.

While most people who have been sick with H1N1 have recovered without needing medical treatment, hospitalizations and deaths from infection with this virus have occurred. About 70 percent of people who have been hospitalized with this H1N1 virus have had one or more medical conditions previously recognized as for high risk of serious seasonal flu-related complications.

Groups at High Risk
The information analyzed by CDC supports the conclusion that 2009 H1N1 flu has caused greater disease burden in people younger than 25 years of age. At this time, there are relatively fewer cases and deaths reported in people 65 years and older, which is unusual when compared with seasonal flu. However, pregnancy and other previously recognized high risk medical conditions from seasonal influenza appear to be associated with increased risk of complications from H1N1. These underlying conditions include asthma, diabetes, suppressed immune systems, heart disease, kidney disease, neurocognitive and neuromuscular disorders and pregnancy.

Young children are also at high risk of serious complications from H1N1, just as they are from seasonal flu. And while people 65 and older are the least likely to be infected with H1N1 flu, if they get sick, they are also at high risk of developing serious complications from their illness. CDC laboratory studies have shown that no children and very few adults younger than 60 years old have existing antibody to H1N1 flu virus; however, about one-third of adults older than 60 may have antibodies against this virus. It is unknown how much, if any, protection may be afforded against 2009 H1N1 flu by any existing antibody.

High risk groups for H1N1 influenza complications include:
- Children younger than 5, but especially children younger than 2 years old
- Adults 65 years of age and older

- Pregnant women

People who have medical conditions including:
- Asthma
- Neurological and neurodevelopmental conditions [including disorders of the brain, spinal cord, peripheral nerve, and muscle such as cerebral palsy, epilepsy (seizure disorders), stroke, intellectual disability (mental retardation), moderate to severe developmental delay, muscular dystrophy, or spinal cord injury].
- Chronic lung disease (such as chronic obstructive pulmonary disease [COPD] and cystic fibrosis)
- Heart disease (such as congenital heart disease, congestive heart failure and coronary artery disease)
- Blood disorders (such as sickle cell disease)
- Endocrine disorders (such as diabetes mellitus)
- Kidney disorders
- Liver disorders
- Metabolic disorders (such as inherited metabolic disorders and mitochondrial disorders)
- Weakened immune system due to disease or medication (such as people with HIV or AIDS, or cancer, or those on chronic steroids)

Young children are less likely to have typical flu symptoms (fever and cough) and infants may have fever and lethargy, and may not have cough or other respiratory symptoms or signs.

Pregnant women who get sick with H1N1 can have serious health problems. They can get sicker than other people who get the flu. Some pregnant women sick with H1N1 have had early labor and severe pneumonia. Some have died. If you are pregnant and have symptoms of the flu, take it very seriously. Call your doctor right away for advice. Adverse pregnancy outcomes have been reported following previous influenza pandemics, with increased rates of spontaneous abortion and preterm birth reported, especially among women with pneumonia. Evidence indicates that pregnancy increases the risk for flu complications for the mother and might increase the risk for other pregnancy related complications.

Symptoms

The symptoms of H1N1 in people are similar to the symptoms of regular human flu and include fever, cough, sore throat, body aches, headache, chills, and fatigue. Some people have also reported diarrhea and vomiting. Like seasonal flu, H1N1 flu may cause a worsening of underlying chronic medical conditions. And like other types of flu viruses, H1N1 is especially dangerous for those with already compromised health conditions, including the elderly.

In children, emergency warning signs that need urgent medical attention include:
- Fast breathing or trouble breathing
- Bluish skin color
- Not drinking enough fluids
- Not waking up or not interacting
- Being so irritable that the child does not want to be held
- Flu-like symptoms improve but then return with fever and worse cough
- Fever with a rash

In adults, emergency warning signs that need urgent medical attention include:
- Difficulty breathing or shortness of breath
- Pain or pressure in the chest or abdomen
- Sudden dizziness

- Confusion
- Severe or persistent vomiting

Transmission

Influenza viruses can be directly transmitted from pigs to people and from people to pigs. Human infection with flu viruses from pigs are most likely to occur when people are in close proximity to infected pigs, such as in pig barns and livestock exhibits housing pigs at fairs. Human-to-human transmission of swine flu can also occur. This is thought to occur in the same way as seasonal flu occurs in people, which is mainly person-to-person transmission through coughing or sneezing of people infected with the influenza virus.

The best advice to prevent contraction of the disease is to get an H1N1 vaccine, avoid people with the flu, stay home if you have any kind of flu, and wash your hands frequently.

Infected people may be able to infect others beginning one day before symptoms develop and up to seven or more days after becoming sick. That means that you may be able to pass on the flu to someone else before you know you are sick. Conversely, you may be able to contract the virus from someone who does not yet show symptoms of illness.

Flu viruses are spread mainly from person to person through coughing or sneezing of people with influenza. Transmission of the virus requires close contact between people because droplets do not remain suspended in the air and generally travel only a short distance (less than three feet) through the air.

H1N1 flu can be spread when a person touches something that is contaminated with the virus and then touches his or her eyes, nose, or mouth. Droplets from a cough or sneeze of an infected person move through the air. H1N1 flu can be spread when a person touches respiratory droplets from another person on a surface like a desk and then touches their own eyes, mouth, or nose before washing their hands. Since this is a new virus in humans, transmission from infected persons to close contacts is common. All respiratory secretions and bodily fluids (diarrheal stool) should be considered potentially infectious.

People with H1N1 infection should be considered potentially contagious as long as they are symptomatic and for up to seven days following illness onset. Children, especially younger children, might potentially be contagious for longer periods.

We know that some viruses and bacteria can live two hours or longer on surfaces like cafeteria tables, doorknobs, and desks. Frequent hand washing will help you reduce the chance of getting swine flu contamination from these common surfaces.

Swine flu viruses are not spread by food. You cannot get swine influenza from eating pork or pork products. Eating properly handled and cooked pork products is safe.

Breastfeeding Considerations
Infants who are not breastfeeding are particularly vulnerable to infection and hospitalization for severe respiratory illness.

If a woman is ill, she should continue breastfeeding and increase feeding frequency. If maternal illness prevents safe feeding at the breast, but pumping is still possible, it should be pursued. The risk for H1N1 transmission through breast milk is unknown.

However, reports of transmission with seasonal flu infection are rare.

Expressed milk should be used for infants too ill to feed at the breast. Antiviral medication treatment or prophylaxis is not a contraindication for breastfeeding.

Diagnosing H1N1

To diagnose swine influenza A infection, a respiratory specimen would generally need to be collected within the first four to five days of illness (when an infected person is most likely to be shedding virus). However, some persons, especially children, may shed virus for ten days or longer. Identification of H1N1 influenza A virus requires sending the specimen to the CDC for laboratory testing.

Test Kits
Immediately after an emergency had been declared by the Secretary of Health and Human Services over of the 2009 H1N1 outbreak, the Food and Drug Administration (FDA) authorized the emergency use of Swine Influenza Test Kits.

Though there is a very small chance that this test can give a result that is wrong (false positive), it is not likely. If a test result from this test is positive, a doctor will decide how to care for the patient based on results as well as other factors like the patient's age and overall health.

Treatment

If you live in areas where swine flu cases have been identified, and you become ill with influenza-like symptoms, including fever, body aches, runny nose, sore throat, nausea, vomiting, or diarrhea, contact your health care provider, particularly if you are worried about your symptoms. Avoid contact with other people as much as possible to keep from spreading your illness to others. Wear a dust mask when in public and wash your hand frequently.

Antiviral Drugs

The CDC recommends the use of Tamiflu or Relenza for the treatment and/or prevention of infection. Antiviral drugs are prescription medicines (pills, liquid, or an inhaler) that fight against the flu by keeping flu viruses from reproducing in your body. If you get sick, antiviral drugs can make your illness milder and make you feel better faster. They may also prevent serious influenza complications. Influenza antiviral drugs work best when started soon after illness onset (within two 2 days), but treatment with antiviral drugs should still be considered after 48 hours of symptom onset, particularly for hospitalized patients or people at high risk for influenza-related complications.

These medications must be prescribed by a health care professional. Influenza antiviral drugs only work against influenza viruses—they will not help treat or prevent symptoms caused by infection from other viruses that can cause symptoms similar to the flu.

The CDC recommends the use of oseltamivir or zanamivir for the treatment and/or prevention of infection with swine influenza viruses.

- Oseltamivir (brand name Tamiflu®) is approved to both treat and prevent influenza A and B virus infection in people one year of age and older.
- Zanamivir (brand name Relenza®) is approved to treat influenza A and B virus infection in people seven years and older and to prevent influenza A and B virus infection in people five years and older.

Recommendations for using antiviral drugs for treatment or prevention of swine influenza will change as more is learned about this new virus. Additional therapy such as antibiotics may be used at the doctor's discretion depending on the patients symptoms.

For hospitalized patients with severe pneumonia requiring intensive care unit admission, menthicillin resistent *Staphylococcus aureus* (MRSA) infection is possible and may need to be treated. For more on MRSA, see Chapter 5.

H1N1 Vaccination

A flu vaccine is the single best way to protect against influenza illness. There is a seasonal flu vaccine to protect against seasonal flu viruses and an H1N1 vaccine to protect against the H1N1 virus. About two weeks after vaccination, antibodies that provide protection against the infection will develop in the body.

The ability of a flu vaccine to protect a person depends on the age and health status of the person receiving it as well as the similarity between the viruses in the vaccine and those in circulation. CDC analyzes circulating influenza viruses on an ongoing basis to determine how closely matched they are to vaccine viruses.

Though the H1N1 vaccine is made using the same processes and facilities used to make the currently licensed seasonal influenza vaccines, the current H1N1 vaccine does not protect against seasonal flu viruses.

Getting Vaccinated

Vaccination should begin as soon as it is available and continue throughout the season into December, January, and beyond. This is because the timing and duration of flu activity can vary. Flu seasons can last as late as April or May. By early October 2009, extensive H1N1 flu activity was reported in the United States. It's possible that there may be waves of H1N1 activity during flu season that hit communities more than once over the course of the season.

Vaccine is available in a combination of settings such as vaccination clinics organized by local health departments, healthcare provider offices, schools, and other private settings, such as pharmacies and workplaces.

While H1N1 viruses are likely to be the most common cause of influenza this season, the seasonal influenza viruses will also circulate and the CDC continues to recommend that people get a seasonal flu vaccine to protect against seasonal flu viruses.

Who Should Get Vaccinated
When vaccine is first available, programs and providers administer it to people in the following five categories (order of groups does not indicate priority)
- pregnant women
- people who live with or provide care for infants younger than six months (e.g., parents, siblings, and day care providers)
- health care and emergency medical services personnel
- people six months through 24 years of age (especially those with higher risk for influenza-related complications like children younger than five years and those who have high risk medical conditions)
- people 25 years through 64 years of age who have certain medical conditions that put them at higher risk for influenza-related complications

No shortage of H1N1 vaccine is expected, but availability and demand can be unpredictable and initially the vaccine may be available in limited quantities.

Once the demand for vaccine for the target groups is met at the local level, programs and providers begin vaccinating everyone from the ages of 25 through 64 years.

Vaccine Side Effects

The same side effects typically associated with the seasonal flu vaccine are expected with the H1N1 vaccine. They are:

H1N1 flu shot: The viruses in the flu shot are killed (inactivated), so you cannot get the flu from a flu shot. Some minor side effects that could occur are:
- Soreness, redness, or swelling where the shot was given
- Fever (low grade)
- Aches

If these problems occur, they begin soon after the shot, are usually mild, and usually last one to two days. Almost all people who receive influenza vaccine have no serious problems from it. However, on rare occasions, flu vaccination can cause serious problems, such as severe allergic reactions.

H1N1 nasal spray: The viruses in the nasal-spray vaccine are weakened and do not cause severe symptoms often associated with influenza illness. (In clinical studies, transmission of vaccine viruses to close contacts has occurred only rarely.) In children, side effects can include:
- runny nose
- wheezing
- headache
- vomiting
- muscle aches

- fever

In adults, side effects can include
- runny nose
- headache
- sore throat
- cough

Egg Allergies

People who are allergic to eggs might be at risk for allergic reactions from influenza vaccines, including the H1N1 vaccine. People who have had any of the following symptoms or experiences should consult with a doctor or other medical professional before considering any influenza vaccination:
- hives or swelling of the lips or tongue
- acute respiratory distress (trouble breathing) after eating eggs
- documented hypersensitivity to eggs, including those who have had asthma related to egg exposure at their workplace or other allergic responses to egg protein

Because children with severe asthma are at high risk of serious complications from influenza, a regimen has been developed for giving influenza vaccine to children with severe asthma and egg hypersensitivity.

Multiple Vaccinations

Inactivated H1N1 vaccine can be administered at the same visit as any other vaccine, including pneumococcal polysaccharide vaccine. Live H1N1 vaccine can be administered at the same visit as any other live or inactivated vaccine EXCEPT seasonal live attenuated influenza vaccine.

Prior Flu-like Illnesses

The symptoms of influenza are similar to those caused by many other viruses. Therefore, if you were ill but do not know if you had H1N1, you should get vaccinated if your doctor recommends it. If you have had H1N1 flu, as confirmed by an official RT-PCR test, you should have some immunity against the current circulation of H1N1 flu and can choose not to get the vaccine. However, vaccination of a person with some existing immunity to will not be harmful.

Vaccination or any other immunity from H1N1 will not provide protection against seasonal influenza. All people who want protection from seasonal flu should still get their seasonal influenza vaccine.

Who Should Not Be Vaccinated

There are some people who should not get any flu vaccine without first consulting a physician. These include:

- People who have a severe allergy to chicken eggs.
- People who have had a severe reaction to an influenza vaccination.
- People who developed Guillain-Barré syndrome (GBS) within six weeks of getting an influenza vaccine previously.
- Children younger than six months of age (influenza vaccine is not approved for this age group)
- People with a moderate-to-severe illness with a fever (they should wait until they recover to get vaccinated)

Alternative Prevention

If you cannot be vaccinated, there are everyday actions that can help prevent the spread of H1N1. First and most important: wash your hands. Try to stay in good general health. Get plenty of sleep, be physically active, manage your stress, drink plenty of fluids, and eat nutritious food. Try not touch surfaces that may be contaminated with the flu virus. Avoid close contact with people who are sick.

Influenza antiviral drugs can be used to prevent influenza when they are given to a person who is not ill, but who has been or may be near a person with swine flu. When used to prevent the flu, antiviral drugs are about 70% to 90% effective. When used for prevention, the number of days that they should be used will vary depending on a person's particular situation.

Take these everyday steps to protect your health:
- Wash your hands often with soap and water, especially after you cough or sneeze. Alcohol-based hand cleaners are also effective.
- Avoid touching your eyes, nose, or mouth. Germs spread this way.
- Try to avoid close contact with sick people.
- If you get sick with influenza, the CDC recommends that you stay home from work or school and limit contact with others to keep from infecting them.

If you are sick, limit your contact with other people as much as possible. Do not go to work or school if ill. Cover your mouth and nose with a tissue when coughing or sneezing. It may prevent those around you from getting sick. Put your used tissue in the waste basket. Cover your cough or sneeze if you do not have a tissue. Then, clean your hands, and do so every time you cough or sneeze.

Washing your hands often will help protect you from germs. Wash with soap and water, or clean with alcohol-based hand cleaner. When you wash your hands with soap and warm water, wash for

15 to 20 seconds. When soap and water are not available, alcohol-based disposable hand wipes or gel sanitizers may be used. You can find them in most supermarkets and drugstores. If using gel, rub your hands until the gel is dry. The gel doesn't need water to work; the alcohol in it kills the germs on your hands. Lotions labeled "anti-bacterial" kill bacteria only. Because H1N1 is a virus, stick to alcohol based agents and those labeled "anti-*microbial*."

Caring for a Person with H1N1

H1N1 can cause a wide range of symptoms, including fever, cough, sore throat, body aches, headache, chills, and fatigue. People with H1N1 can also have vomiting and diarrhea. Like seasonal flu, swine flu in humans can vary in severity from mild to severe. Severe disease with pneumonia, respiratory failure, and even death is possible with swine flu infection. Certain groups might be more likely to develop a severe illness, such as persons with chronic medical conditions. Sometimes bacterial infections may occur at the same time as or after infection and lead to pneumonias, ear infections, or sinus infections.

The following information can help you provide safer care at home for sick persons during a flu pandemic.

People with H1N1 swine flu who are cared for at home should:
- check with their health care provider about any special care they might need if they are pregnant or have a health condition such as diabetes, heart disease, asthma, or emphysema
- check with their health care provider about whether they should take antiviral medications
- stay home for seven days after the start of illness and fever is gone
- get plenty of rest

- drink clear fluids (such as water, broth, sports drinks, electrolyte beverages for infants) to keep from being dehydrated
- cover coughs and sneezes. Clean hands with soap and water or an alcohol-based hand rub often and especially after using tissues and after coughing or sneezing into hands.
- avoid close contact with others—do not go to work or school while ill
- be watchful for emergency warning signs (see pg 46) that might indicate you need to seek medical attention

Medications to Lessen Symptoms of the Flu

NOTICE: *Check with your healthcare provider or pharmacist for correct, safe use of medications.*

Antiviral medications can sometimes lessen flu symptoms, but require a prescription. Most people do not need antiviral drugs to fully recover from the flu. However, persons at higher risk for severe complications, or those with severe illness who require hospitalization, might benefit from antiviral medications. Antiviral medications are available for persons one year of age and older. Ask your healthcare provider whether you need antiviral medication.

Influenza infections can lead to or occur with bacterial infections. Therefore, some people will also need to take antibiotics. More severe or prolonged illness or illness that seems to get better, but then gets worse again may be an indication that a person has a bacterial infection. Check with your healthcare provider if you have concerns.

Warning! Do *not* give aspirin (acetylsalicylic acid) to children or teenagers who have the flu; this can cause a rare but serious illness called Reye's syndrome.

- Check ingredient labels on over-the-counter cold and flu medications to see if they contain aspirin.
- Teenagers with the flu can take medicines *without* aspirin, such as acetaminophen (Tylenol®) and ibuprofen (Advil®, Motrin®, Nuprin®), to relieve symptoms.
- Children younger than two years of age should not be given over-the-counter cold medications without first speaking with a healthcare provider.
- The safest care for flu symptoms in children younger than two years of age is using a cool-mist humidifier and a suction bulb to help clear away mucus.
- Fevers and aches can be treated with acetaminophen (Tylenol®) or ibuprofen (Advil®, Motrin®, Nuprin®) or nonsteroidal anti-inflammatory drugs (NSAIDS). Examples of these kinds of medications include:

Generic Name	Brand Name(s)
Acetaminophen	Tylenol®
Ibuprofen	Advil®, Motrin®, Nuprin®
Naproxen	Aleve

- Over-the-counter cold and flu medications used according to the package instructions may help lessen some symptoms such as cough and congestion. However, these medications will *not* lessen how infectious a person is.
- Check the ingredients on the package label to see if the medication already contains acetaminophen or ibuprofen before taking additional doses of these medications—don't double dose! Patients with kidney disease or stomach

problems should check with their health care provider before taking any NSAIDS.

- Check with your health care provider or pharmacist if you are taking other over-the-counter or prescription medications not related to the flu.

When to Seek Emergency Medical Care
Get medical care right away if the sick person at home:
- has difficulty breathing or chest pain
- has purple or blue discoloration of the lips
- is vomiting and unable to keep liquids down
- has signs of dehydration such as dizziness when standing, absence of urination, or in infants, a lack of tears when they cry
- has seizures (for example, uncontrolled convulsions)
- is less responsive than normal or becomes confused

Reduce the Spread of Flu in the Home

When providing care to a household member who is sick, the most important ways to protect yourself and others who are not sick are to:
- keep the sick person away from other people as much as possible (see "placement of the sick person at home")
- remind the sick person to cover their coughs, and clean their hands with soap and water or an alcohol-based hand rub often, especially after coughing and/or sneezing.
- have everyone in the household clean their hands often, using soap and water or an alcohol-based hand rub
- ask your healthcare provider if household contacts of the sick person—particularly those contacts who may have chronic health conditions—should take antiviral medications such as oseltamivir (Tamiflu®) or zanamivir (Relenza®) to prevent the flu.

Placement of the sick person

- Keep the sick person in a room separate from the common areas of the house. (For example, a spare bedroom with its own bathroom, if that's possible.) Keep the sickroom door closed.
- Unless necessary for medical care, persons with the flu should not leave the home when they have a fever or during the time that they are most likely to spread their infection to others (seven days after onset of symptoms in adults. Children may pass the virus for longer than seven days).
- If persons with the flu need to leave the home (for example, for medical care), they should cover their nose and mouth when coughing or sneezing and wear a loose-fitting (surgical) mask if available.
- Have the sick person wear a surgical mask if they need to be in a common area of the house near other persons.
- If possible, sick persons should use a separate bathroom. This bathroom should be cleaned daily with household disinfectant (see below).

Protect other persons in the home

- The sick person should not have visitors other than caregivers. A phone call is safer than a visit.
- If possible, have only one adult in the home take care of the sick person.
- Avoid having pregnant women care for the sick person. (Pregnant women are at increased risk of flu-related complications and immunity can be suppressed during pregnancy).
- All persons in the household should clean their hands with soap and water or an alcohol-based hand rub frequently, including after every contact with the sick person or the person's room or bathroom.

- Use paper towels for drying hands after hand washing or dedicate cloth towels to each person in the household. For example, have different colored towels for each person.
- If possible, consideration should be given to maintaining good ventilation in shared household areas (e.g., keeping windows open in restrooms, kitchen, bathroom, etc.).
- Antivirals can be used to prevent the flu, so check with your healthcare provider to see if some persons in the home should use antiviral medications.

If you are the caregiver
- Avoid being face-to-face with the sick person.
- When holding small children who are sick, place their chin on your shoulder so that they will not cough in your face.
- Caregivers might catch flu from the person they are caring for and then the caregiver might be able to spread the flu to others before the caregiver shows symptoms. Therefore, the caregiver should wear a mask when they leave their home to keep from spreading flu to others in case they are in the early stages of infection.
- Talk to your health care provider about taking antiviral medication to prevent the caregiver from getting the flu.
- Monitor yourself and household members for flu symptoms and contact a health care provider if symptoms occur.

Using Facemasks or Respirators
- Avoid close contact (less than about six feet away) with the sick person as much as possible.
- If you must have close contact with the sick person (for example, hold a sick infant), spend the least amount of time possible in close contact and try to wear a facemask (for example, surgical mask) or N95 disposable respirator.

- An N95 respirator that fits snugly on your face can filter out small particles that can be inhaled around the edges of a facemask, but compared with a facemask it is harder to breathe through an N95 mask for long periods of time.
- Facemasks and respirators may be purchased at a pharmacy, building supply or hardware store.
- Wear an N95 respirator if you help a sick person with respiratory treatments using a nebulizer or inhaler, as directed by their doctor. Respiratory treatments should be performed in a separate room away from common areas of the house when at all possible.
- Used facemasks and N95 respirators should be taken off and placed immediately in the regular trash so they don't touch anything else.
- Avoid re-using disposable facemasks and N95 respirators if possible. If a reusable fabric facemask is used, it should be laundered with normal laundry detergent and tumble-dried in a hot dryer.
- After you take off a facemask or N95 respirator, clean your hands with soap and water or an alcohol-based hand sanitizer.

Household Cleaning, Laundry, and Waste Disposal
- Throw away tissues and other disposable items used by the sick person in the trash. Wash your hands after touching used tissues and similar waste.
- Keep surfaces (especially bedside tables, surfaces in the bathroom, and toys for children) clean by wiping them down with a household disinfectant according to directions on the product label.
- Wash linens (such as bed sheets and towels) by using household laundry soap and tumble dry on a hot setting. Avoid "hugging" laundry prior to washing it to prevent contaminating yourself. Clean your hands with soap and

water or alcohol-based hand rub right after handling dirty laundry.

- Eating utensils should be washed either in a dishwasher or by hand with water and soap.

Facemask and Respirator Use

Facemasks are disposable masks cleared by the U.S. Food and Drug Administration (FDA) for use as medical devices. This includes facemasks labeled as surgical, dental, medical procedure, isolation, or laser masks. Such facemasks have several designs. One type is affixed to the head with two ties, conforms to the face with the aid of a flexible adjustment for the nose bridge, and may be flat/pleated or duck-billed in shape. Another type of facemask is pre-molded, adheres to the head with a single elastic band, and has a flexible adjustment for the nose bridge. A third type is flat/pleated and affixes to the head with ear loops. Facemasks cleared by the FDA for use as medical devices have been determined to have specific levels of protection from penetration of blood and body fluids.

An N95 respirator is a higher filtering face piece respirator certified by the U.S. National Institute for Occupational Safety and Health (NIOSH).

Information on the effectiveness of facemasks and respirators for the control of influenza in community settings is extremely limited. Thus, it is difficult to assess their potential effectiveness in controlling H1N1 transmission in these settings. In the absence of clear scientific data, the recommendations below have been developed on the basis of public health judgment and the historical use of facemasks and respirators in other settings.

In areas with confirmed human cases of swine flu, the risk for infection can be reduced through a combination of actions. No single action will provide complete protection, but an approach combining the following steps can help decrease the likelihood of transmission. These actions include frequent hand washing, covering coughs, and having ill persons stay home, except to seek medical care, and minimize contact with others in the household. Additional measures that can limit transmission of a new influenza strain include voluntary home quarantine of members of households with confirmed or probable influenza cases, reduction of unnecessary social contacts, and avoidance whenever possible of crowded settings.

When it is absolutely necessary to enter a crowded setting or to have close contact with persons who might be ill, the time spent in that setting should be as short as possible. If used correctly, facemasks and respirators may help reduce the risk of getting the flu, but they should be used along with other preventive measures, such as avoiding close contact and maintaining good hand hygiene.

The use of facemasks or respirators should be considered as follows:
1. Whenever possible, rather than relying on the use of facemasks or respirators, close contact with people who might be ill and being in crowded settings should be avoided.
2. Facemasks should be considered for use by individuals who enter crowded settings, both to protect their nose and mouth from other people's coughs and to reduce the wearers' likelihood of coughing on others; the time spent in crowded settings should be as short as possible.
3. Respirators should be considered for use by individuals for whom close contact with an infectious person is unavoidable. This can include selected individuals who

must care for a sick person (e.g., family member with a respiratory infection) at home.

For Medical Personnel

The infectious period for a confirmed case of swine influenza A (H1N1) virus infection is defined as one day prior to the case's illness onset to seven days after onset.

Close contact is defined as: within about six feet of an ill person who is a confirmed or suspected case of swine-origin influenza A (H1N1) virus infection during the case's infectious period. Acute respiratory illness is defined as recent onset of at least two of the following: rhinorrhea or nasal congestion, sore throat, cough (with or without fever or feverishness)

Clinicians should suspect swine-origin influenza A (H1N1) in persons with an acute febrile respiratory illness who
- Have had close contact with a person who is a swine-origin influenza confirmed case *or*
- Traveled to a community in the United States or internationally where there are one or more confirmed swine-origin influenza cases (Updated information about areas with confirmed human cases of swine-origin influenza A (H1N1) can be found at www.cdc.gov/h1n1flu/investigation.htm.) *or*
- Reside in a community where there are confirmed swine-origin influenza A (H1N1) cases.

Patients with uncomplicated disease due to confirmed swine-origin influenza A (H1N1) virus infection have experienced fever, headache, upper respiratory tract symptoms (cough, sore throat, rhinorrhea), myalgia, fatigue, vomiting, or diarrhea.

Clinicians who suspect H1N1 infections in humans should obtain a nasopharyngeal swab from the patient, place the swab in a viral transport medium, refrigerate the specimen, and then contact their state or local health department to facilitate transport and timely diagnosis at a state public health laboratory. The CDC requests that state public health laboratories promptly send all influenza A specimens that cannot be subtyped to the CDC, Influenza Division, Virus Surveillance and Diagnostics Branch Laboratory.

Persons with febrile respiratory illness should be advised to stay home from work or school to avoid spreading infections (including influenza and other respiratory illnesses) to others in their communities. In addition, frequent hand washing can lessen the spread of respiratory illness.

There is insufficient information to date about clinical complications of this variant of swine-origin influenza A (H1N1) virus infection. Among persons infected with previous variants of swine influenza virus, clinical syndromes have ranged from mild respiratory illness, to lower respiratory tract illness, dehydration, or pneumonia. Deaths caused by swine influenza have occurred. Clinicians should expect complications to be similar to seasonal influenza: exacerbation of underlying chronic medical conditions, upper respiratory tract disease (sinusitis, otitis media, croup) lower respiratory tract disease (pneumonia, bronchiolitis, status asthmaticus), cardiac (myocarditis, pericarditis), musculoskeletal (myositis, rhabdomyolysis), neurologic (acute and post-infectious encephalopathy, encephalitis, febrile seizures, status epilepticus), toxic shock syndrome, and secondary bacterial pneumonia with or without sepsis.

Treatment

The swine-origin influenza virus is susceptible to both oseltamivir and zanamivir. It is resistant to amantadine and rimantadine. Additional therapy such as antibacterial agents, should be used at the discretion of the clinicians given the patients clinical presentation. For antibacterial treatment of pneumonia, clinical guidance for community-acquired pneumonia should be followed and can be accessed at: www.journals.uchicago.edu.

For hospitalized patients with severe community-acquired pneumonia (CAP) requiring intensive care unit admission, menthicillin-resistent *Staphylococcus aureus* (MRSA) infection should be suspected and treated empirically in addition to other causes of CAP if they have 1) necrotizing or cavitary infiltrates or 2) empyema.

Pregnant Women

Evidence that influenza can be more severe in pregnant women comes from observations during previous pandemics and from studies among pregnant women who had seasonal influenza. An excess of influenza-associated excess deaths among pregnant women were reported during the pandemics of 1918-1919 and 1957-1958. Adverse pregnancy outcomes have been reported following previous influenza pandemics, with increased rates of spontaneous abortion and preterm birth reported, especially among women with pneumonia. Case reports and several epidemiologic studies conducted during interpandemic periods also indicate that pregnancy increases the risk for influenza complications for the mother and might increase the risk for adverse perinatal outcomes or delivery complications.

Clinical Presentation

Pregnant women with swine influenza would be expected to present with typical acute respiratory illness (e.g., cough, sore throat, rhinorrhea) and fever or feverishness. Many pregnant women will go on to have a typical course of uncomplicated influenza. However, for some pregnant women, illness might progress rapidly, and might be complicated by secondary bacterial infections including pneumonia. Fetal distress associated with severe maternal illness can occur. Pregnant women who have suspected swine influenza A (H1N1) virus infection should be tested, and specimens from women who have unsubtypeable influenza A virus infections should have specimens sent to the state public health laboratory for additional testing to identify swine influenza A (H1N1).

Treatment and Chemoprophylaxis
The currently circulating swine influenza A (H1N1) virus is sensitive to the neuraminidase inhibitor antiviral medications zanamivir (Relenza®) and oseltamivir (Tamiflu®), but is resistant to the adamantane antiviral medications, amantadine (Symmetrel®) and rimantadine (Flumadine®). Pregnant women who meet current case-definitions for confirmed, probable, or suspected swine influenza A (H1N1) infection should receive empiric antiviral treatment. Pregnant women who are close contacts with persons with suspected, probable, or confirmed cases of swine influenza A (H1N1) should receive chemoprophylaxis.

As is recommended for other persons who are treated, antiviral treatment with zanamivir or oseltamivir should be initiated as soon as possible after the onset of influenza symptoms, with benefits expected to be greatest if started within 48 hours of onset based on date from studies of seasonal influenza. However, some data from studies on seasonal influenza indicate benefit for hospitalized patients even if treatment is started more than 48 hours after onset. Recommended duration of treatment is five days, and for chemoprophylaxis is ten days. Oseltamivir and zanamivir treatment and chemoprophylaxis regimens recommended for pregnant women are the same as those recommended for adults who have seasonal influenza.

One of the more well-studied adverse effects of influenza is its associated hyperthermia. Studies have shown that maternal hyperthermia during the first trimester doubles the risk of neural tube defects and may be associated with other birth defects and adverse outcomes. Limited data suggest that the risk for birth defects associated with fever might be mitigated by antipyretic medications or multivitamins that contain folic acid. Maternal fever during labor has been shown to be a risk factor for adverse neonatal and developmental outcomes, including neonatal seizures, encephalopathy, cerebral palsy, and neonatal death. Even though distinguishing the effects of the cause of fever from the hyperthermia itself is difficult, fever in pregnant women should be treated because of the risk that hyperthermia appears to pose to the fetus. Acetaminophen appears to be the best option for treatment of fever during pregnancy although data on this common exposure are also limited.

Pregnancy should not be considered a contraindication to oseltamivir or zanamivir use. Pregnant women might be at higher risk for severe complications from swine influenza, and the benefits of treatment or chemoprophylaxis with zanamivir or oseltamivir likely outweigh the theoretical risks of antiviral use. Oseltamivir and zanamivir are "Pregnancy Category C" medications, indicating that no clinical studies have been conducted to assess the safety of these medications for pregnant women. Because of the unknown effects of influenza antiviral drugs on pregnant women and their fetuses, oseltamivir or zanamivir should be used during pregnancy only if the potential benefit justifies the potential risk to the embryo or fetus.

Though a few adverse effects have been reported in pregnant women who took these medications, no relation between the use of these medications and those adverse events has been established. Because zanamivir is an inhaled medication and has less systemic absorption, some experts prefer zanamivir for use in pregnant women when feasible. Because of its systemic activity, oseltamivir is preferred for treatment of pregnant women. The drug of choice for prophylaxis is less clear. Zanamivir may be preferable because of its limited systemic absorption; however, respiratory complications that may be associated with zanamivir, because of its inhaled route of administration, need to be considered, especially in women at risk for respiratory problems.

Patients with Cardiovascular Disease

Patients with chronic cardiovascular disease and cerebrovascular disease (CVD) are at increased risk of experiencing an acute exacerbation of disease during influenza epidemics. Patients with CVD risk factors such as hypertension, smoking, obesity, and family history of premature heart disease might be considered for priority care over healthy individuals but not before health care providers, the very young, elderly people, and the ill.

Health care providers should be aware that influenza might produce increased numbers of cardiovascular events, leading to increased hospitalizations and use of resources to treat acute coronary events, heart failure, and stroke. Consideration should be given for having adequate supplies of commonly used cardiovascular medications for prevention and treatment of cardiovascular events.

What is Being Done

The CDC has implemented its emergency response. The agency's goals are to reduce transmission and illness severity, and provide information to help health care providers, public health officials, and the public address the challenges posed by the new virus. CDC continues to issue new interim guidance for clinicians and public health professionals. In addition, CDC's Division of the Strategic National Stockpile (SNS) continues to send antiviral drugs, personal protective equipment, and respiratory protection devices to all 50 states and U.S. territories to help them respond to the outbreak.

Epidemiological Investigations

The CDC works very closely with state and local officials in areas where human cases of H1N1 infections have been identified. In California and Texas, where EpiAid teams have been deployed, many epidemiological activities are taking place or planned including:

- Active surveillance in the counties where infections in humans have been identified;
- Studies of health care workers who were exposed to patients infected with the virus to see if they became infected;
- Studies of households and other contacts of people who were confirmed to have been infected to see if they became infected;
- Study of a public high school where three confirmed human cases of influenza A (H1N1) of swine origin occurred to see if anyone became infected and how much contact they had with a confirmed case;
- Study to see how long a person with the virus infection sheds the virus.

- Links to non-federal organizations are provided solely as a service to users. These links do not constitute an endorsement of these organizations or their programs by CDC or the federal government, and none should be inferred. CDC is not responsible for the content of the individual organization Web pages found at these links.

Common Questions

What is H1N1 (swine flu)?

H1N1 (referred to as "swine flu" early on) is a new influenza virus causing illness in people. This new virus was first detected in people in April 2009 in the United States. By early May, the virus reached worldwide pandemic levels. This virus is spreading from person-to-person, in much the same way that regular seasonal influenza viruses spread.

Is this new H1N1 virus contagious?

The CDC has determined that this new H1N1 virus is contagious and is spreading from human to human.

What are the signs and symptoms of H1N1 in people?

The symptoms are similar to the symptoms of regular human flu and include fever, cough, sore throat, body aches, headache, chills, and fatigue. A significant number of people who have been infected with this virus also have reported diarrhea and vomiting. Also, like seasonal flu, severe illnesses and death have occurred as a result of illness associated with this virus.

How severe is illness associated with H1N1 virus?

It's not known at this time how severe this virus will be in the general population. The CDC is studying the medical histories of people who have been infected with this virus to determine whether some people may be at greater risk from infection, serious illness, or hospitalization from the virus. There are certain people that are at higher risk of serious flu-related complications. This includes young children, pregnant women, people with chronic medical conditions, and people 65 and older. The CDC also is conducting laboratory studies to see if certain people might have natural immunity to this virus, depending on their age.

Why is H1N1 virus sometimes called "swine flu"?

This virus was originally referred to as "swine flu" because laboratory testing showed that many of the genes in this new virus were very similar to influenza viruses that normally occur in pigs. Further study has shown that this new virus is very different from what normally circulates in pigs.

Do pigs carry this virus and can I catch this virus from a pig?

At this time, there is no evidence that swine in the United States are infected with this new virus. However, there are flu viruses that commonly cause outbreaks of illness in pigs. Most of the time, these viruses do not infect people, but it is possible for influenza viruses to spread back and forth between pigs and people.

Can I get H1N1 more than once?

Getting infected with any influenza virus, including 2009 H1N1, should cause your body to develop immune resistance to that virus so it's not likely that a person would be infected with the identical influenza virus more than once. (However, people with weakened immune systems might not develop full immunity after infection and might be more likely to get infected with the same influenza virus more than once.) However, it's also possible that a person could have a positive test result for flu infection more than once in an influenza season. This can occur for two reasons:

1. A person may be infected with different influenza viruses (for example, the first time with 2009 H1N1 and the

second time with a regular seasonal flu virus. Most rapid tests cannot distinguish which influenza virus is responsible for the illness. And,

2. Influenza tests can occasionally give false positive and false negative results so it's possible that one of the test results were incorrect. This is more likely to happen when the diagnosis is made with the rapid flu tests. More information about flu diagnosis is available at http://www.cdc.gov/h1n1flu/diagnosis/.

Can I get infected with this new H1N1 virus from eating or preparing pork?

No. H1N1 viruses are not spread by food. You cannot get this new HIN1 virus from eating pork or pork products. Eating properly handled and cooked pork products is safe.

How does H1N1 virus spread?

Spread of H1N1 is happening in the same way that seasonal flu spreads. Flu viruses are spread mainly from person to person through coughing or sneezing by people with influenza. Sometimes people may become infected by touching something with flu viruses on it and then touching their mouth or nose.

Is there a risk from drinking water?

Tap water that has been treated by conventional disinfection processes does not likely pose a risk for transmission of influenza viruses. Current drinking water treatment regulations provide a high degree of protection from viruses. No research has been completed on the susceptibility of the new H1N1 flu virus to conventional drinking water treatment processes. However, recent studies have demonstrated that free chlorine levels typically used in drinking water treatment are adequate to inactivate highly pathogenic H5N1 avian influenza. It is likely that other influenza viruses such as the new H1N1 would also be similarly inactivated by chlorination. To date, there have been no documented human cases of influenza caused by exposure to contaminated drinking water.

Can the virus be spread through water in swimming pools, spas, water parks, interactive fountains, and other treated recreational water venues?

Recreational water that has been treated at recommended disinfectant levels does not likely pose a risk for transmission of influenza viruses. Currently, there are no documented human cases of influenza caused by contaminated swimming pool water. No research has been completed on the susceptibility of the flu virus to chlorine and other disinfectants used in swimming pools, spas, water parks, interactive fountains, and other treated recreational venues. However, recent studies have demonstrated that free chlorine levels recommended by CDC are adequate to disinfect highly pathogenic flu viruses.

Can H1N1 influenza virus be spread at recreational water venues outside of the water?

Yes, recreational water venues are no different than any other group setting. Flu viruses are spread mainly from person to person through coughing or sneezing of people with influenza.

What should I do to keep from getting the flu?

First and most important: get vaccinated. Next, wash your hands. Try to stay in good general health. Get plenty of sleep, be physically active, manage your stress, drink plenty of fluids, and eat nutritious food. Try not to touch surfaces that may be contaminated with the flu virus. Avoid close contact with people who are sick.

Other actions that can help prevent the spread of germs that cause the flu include:

- Cover your nose and mouth with a tissue when you cough or sneeze. Throw the tissue in the trash after you use it.
- Wash your hands often with soap and water, especially after you cough or sneeze. Alcohol-based hand cleaners are also effective.
- Avoid touching your eyes, nose, or mouth. Germs spread this way.
- Try to avoid close contact with sick people.
- Stay home if you are sick for seven days after your symptoms begin or until you have been symptom-free for 24 hours, whichever is longer. This is to keep from infecting others and spreading the virus further.

Be prepared in case you get sick and need to stay home for a week or so; a supply of over-the-counter medicines, alcohol-based hand rubs, tissues and other related items that could be useful and help avoid the need to make trips out in public while you are sick and contagious. Follow public health advice regarding school closures, avoiding crowds, and other social distancing measures.

Will the 2009 H1N1 influenza vaccine contain thimerosal?
The 2009 H1N1 influenza vaccines that FDA is licensing will be manufactured in several formulations. Some will come in multi-dose vials and will contain thimerosal as a preservative to prevent potential contamination after the vial is opened.
Some 2009 H1N1 influenza vaccines will be available in single-dose units, which will not require the use of thimerosal as a preservative. In addition, the live-attenuated version of the vaccine, which is administered through the nose, is produced in single-units and will not contain thimerosal.

Will the benefits of the 2009 H1N1 influenza vaccines outweigh the risks? Is this something I should talk to my healthcare provider about?

Currently the 2009 H1N1 influenza virus seems to be causing serious health outcomes for:

1. healthy young people from birth through age 24;
2. pregnant women; and
3. adults 25 to 64 who have underlying medical conditions.
4. Children, especially those younger than 5 years of age and those who have high risk medical conditions are at increased risk of influenza-related complications.

Seasonal influenza vaccines are highly effective in preventing influenza disease. The expectation is that a vaccine against 2009 H1N1 influenza would probably work in a similar fashion to the seasonal influenza vaccines. CDC and FDA believe that the benefits of vaccination with the 2009 H1N1 influenza vaccine will far outweigh the risks.

Vaccination is the best way to prevent influenza infection and its complications. This is the reason that CDC, national health organizations, and healthcare providers intensively promote vaccination for seasonal influenza, and the reason why so much work was done to have a vaccine available for the 2009 H1N1 influenza virus.

Influenza vaccines do not protect against other viruses that cause respiratory illnesses. Even after you are vaccinated, it is still important to wash your hands well and often, to cover your coughs and sneezes, and to stay home if you are sick.

CDC and FDA encourage you to ask your healthcare provider any questions you may have about the H1N1 influenza vaccine and the seasonal influenza vaccines that will be available during the 2009-2010 influenza season. Your healthcare provider is an excellent source for information on the benefits and risks of vaccination for protection against H1N1 influenza for you, your children, and other family members.

Will there be a possibility of Guillain-Barré Syndrome (GBS) cases following the vaccine?

Guillain-Barré syndrome (GBS) is a rare disease in which the body damages its own nerve cells, causing muscle weakness and sometimes paralysis. It is not fully understood why some people develop GBS, but it is believed that stimulation of the body's immune system may play a role in its development.

Infection with the bacterium Campylobacter jejuni, which can cause diarrhea, is one of the most common risk factors for GBS. People can also develop GBS after having the flu or other infections (such as cytomegalovirus and Epstein Barr virus). On very rare occasions, they may develop GBS in the days or weeks following receiving a vaccination.

In 1976, there was a small risk of GBS following influenza (swine flu) vaccination (approximately 1 additional case per 100,000 people who received the swine flu vaccine). That number of GBS cases was slightly higher than what is normally seen in the population, whether or not people were vaccinated. Since then, numerous studies have been done to evaluate if other flu vaccines were associated with GBS. In most studies, no association was found, but two studies suggested that approximately 1 additional person out of 1 million vaccinated people may be at risk for GBS associated with the seasonal influenza vaccine.

Are there medicines to treat H1N1?

Yes. CDC recommends the use of oseltamivir or zanamivir for the treatment and/or prevention of infection of influenza A (H1N1) viruses. Antiviral drugs are prescription medicines (pills, liquid, or an inhaler) that fight against the flu by keeping flu viruses from reproducing in your body. If you get sick, antiviral drugs can make your illness milder and make you feel better faster. They may also prevent serious flu complications. During the current outbreak, the priority use for influenza antiviral drugs is to treat severe influenza illness.

How long can an infected person spread this virus to others?

At the current time, the CDC believes that this virus has the same properties in terms of spread as seasonal flu viruses. With seasonal flu, studies have shown that people may be contagious from one day before they develop symptoms to up to seven days after they get sick. Children, especially younger children, might potentially be contagious for longer periods. The CDC is studying the virus and its capabilities to try to learn more and will provide more information as it becomes available.

What surfaces are most likely to be sources of contamination?

Germs can be spread when a person touches something that is contaminated with germs and then touches his or her eyes, nose, or mouth. Droplets from a cough or sneeze of an infected person move through the air. Germs can be spread when a person touches respiratory droplets on a surface like a desk, for example, and then touches their own eyes, mouth, or nose before washing their hands.

Studies have shown that influenza virus can survive on surfaces and can infect a person for up to 2-8 hours after being deposited on the surface.

What is the best technique for washing my hands to avoid getting the flu?

Washing your hands often will help protect you from germs. Wash with soap and water or clean with alcohol-based hand cleaner. When you wash your hands with soap and warm water, wash for 15 to 20 seconds. When soap and water are not available, alcohol-based disposable hand wipes or gel sanitizers may be used. You can find them in most supermarkets and drugstores. If using gel, rub your hands until the gel is dry. The gel doesn't need water to work; the alcohol in it kills the germs on your hands.

What should I do if I get sick?

If you live in areas where swine influenza cases have been identified and become ill with influenza-like symptoms, including fever, body aches, runny nose, sore throat, nausea, or vomiting or diarrhea, you may want to contact a health care provider, particularly if you are worried about your symptoms. Your health care provider will determine whether influenza testing or treatment is needed.

If you are sick, you should stay home and avoid contact with other people as much as possible to keep from spreading your illness to others.

What kills influenza virus?

Influenza virus is destroyed by heat (167-212°F [75-100°C]). In addition, several chemical germicides, including chlorine, hydrogen peroxide, detergents (soap), iodophors (iodine-based antiseptics), and alcohols are effective against human influenza viruses if used in proper concentration for a sufficient length of time.

How should waste disposal be handled?

To prevent the spread of influenza virus, it is recommended that tissues and other disposable items used by an infected person be thrown in the trash. Additionally, persons should wash their hands with soap and water after touching used tissues and similar waste.

What household cleaning should be done to prevent the spread of influenza virus?

To prevent the spread of influenza virus, it is important to keep surfaces (especially bedside tables, surfaces in the bathroom, kitchen counters, and toys for children) clean by wiping them down with a household disinfectant according to directions on the product label.

How should linens, eating utensils, and dishes of persons infected with influenza virus be handled?

Linens, eating utensils, and dishes belonging to those who are sick do not need to be cleaned separately, but these items should not be shared without washing thoroughly first. Linens (such as bed sheets and towels) should be washed using household laundry soap and tumbled dry on a hot setting. Individuals should avoid "hugging" laundry prior to washing it to prevent contaminating themselves. Individuals should wash their hands with soap and water or alcohol-based hand rub immediately after handling dirty laundry.

Eating utensils should be washed either in a dishwasher or by hand with water and soap.

Note: Much of this information is based on studies and past experience with seasonal (human) influenza. The CDC believes the information applies to the H1N1 (swine) viruses as well, but studies on this virus are ongoing to learn more about its characteristics.

5

Avian Flu

The biggest concern over avian flu is the possibility that the virus will re-assort in the same way the swine flu did to infect humans more readily. Unlike the current H1N1 flu pandemic, a potential avian flu pandemic could be much more deadly to humans. The information we have from past avian flu outbreaks show that fewer than half of people who become infected survive the disease. The recent H1N1 flu outbreak has demonstrated to scientists just how easy it would be for the avian flu to mutate into a form that could be passed from human to human.

The World Health Organization has reported human cases of avian influenza A (H5N1) in Asia, Africa, the Pacific, Europe, and the Near East. Indonesia and Vietnam have reported the highest number of cases to date. Overall mortality is approximately 60%. The majority of cases have occurred among children and adults aged less than 40 years old. Mortality was highest in cases aged 10-19 years old. Studies have documented the most significant risk factors to be direct contact with sick or dead poultry, wild birds, or visiting a live poultry market.

Most cases have been hospitalized late in their illness with severe respiratory disease. A small number of mild cases have been reported. The latest cumulative numbers of confirmed human cases of avian influenza A/(H5N1) are available on the WHO Avian Influenza website. Despite the high mortality, human cases remain rare to date.

The highly pathogenic avian influenza outbreak in Asia, Europe, the Near East, and Africa is not expected to diminish significantly in the short term. It is likely that the viral infections among domestic poultry have become endemic in certain areas and that sporadic human infections resulting from direct contact with infected poultry and/or wild birds will continue to occur.

Usually, "avian influenza virus" refers to influenza A viruses found chiefly in birds, but infections with these viruses can occur in humans. The risk from avian influenza is generally low to most people because the viruses do not usually infect humans. However, confirmed cases of human infection from several subtypes of avian flu have been reported since 1997.

Most cases of avian flu in humans have resulted from contact with infected poultry (domesticated chicken, ducks, and turkeys) or surfaces contaminated with secretion/excretions from infected birds. The spread of avian flu from one ill person to another has been reported very rarely and has shown not to transmit easily.

Human influenza virus usually refers to those subtypes that spread widely among humans. There are only three known A subtypes of influenza viruses (H1N1, H1N2, and H3N2) currently circulating among humans. It is likely that some genetic parts of current human influenza A viruses came from birds originally. Influenza A viruses are constantly changing, and they might adapt over time to infect and spread among humans. This is the biggest fear and human risk associated with bird flu.

There is little pre-existing natural immunity to this virus in the human population. If it gains the ability for efficient and sustained transmission among humans, an influenza pandemic could result with potentially high rates of illness and death worldwide.

No evidence for genetic reassortment between human and avian influenza A virus genes has been found to date, and there is no evidence of any significant changes to strains to suggest greater transmissibility to humans. Research suggests that the current strains are becoming more capable of causing disease in animals than were earlier strains. One study found that ducks infected with H5N1 virus are now shedding more virus for longer periods without showing symptoms of illness. This finding has implications for the role of ducks in transmitting disease to other birds and possibly to humans as well.

Additionally, other findings have documented infection among pigs in China and Vietnam; discovery of the virus in domestic cats in Germany and Thailand, and detection of viral RNA in domestic cats in Iraq and Austria; infection of dogs in Thailand; and discovery of the viruses in tigers and leopards at zoos in Thailand.

Avian flu strains that emerged in Asia in 2003 continue to evolve and may adapt so that other mammals may be susceptible to infection as well.

Outbreaks of avian fluoccurred among poultry in eight countries in Asia (Cambodia, China, Indonesia, Japan, Laos, South Korea, Thailand, and Vietnam) during late 2003 and early 2004. At that time, more than 100 million birds in the affected countries either died from the disease or were killed in order to try to control the outbreaks. By March 2004, the outbreak was reported to be under control.

Human cases have been reported in Azerbaijan, Bangladesh, Cambodia, China, Djibouti, Egypt, Indonesia, Iraq, Lao People's Democratic Republic, Myanmar, Nigeria, Pakistan, Thailand, Turkey, and Vietnam.

Human Health Risks
Of the few avian influenza viruses that have crossed the species barrier to infect humans, H5N1 has caused the largest number of detected cases of severe disease and death in humans. However, it is possible that only the cases in the most severely ill people are diagnosed and reported.

Of the human cases associated with the recent bird flu outbreaks, more than half of the people infected with the virus have died. Most cases have occurred in previously healthy children and young adults and have resulted from direct or close contact with infected poultry or contaminated surfaces. In general, H5N1 remains a very rare disease in people. The virus does not infect humans easily, and if a person is infected, it is very difficult for the virus to spread to another person.

Nonetheless, because all influenza viruses have the ability to change, scientists are concerned that the avian flu could one day infect humans and spread easily from one person to another. Because these viruses do not commonly infect humans, there is little or no immune protection against them in the human population. If the virus were to gain the capacity to spread easily from person to person, a worldwide influenza pandemic could begin.

No one can predict when a pandemic might occur. However, experts from around the world are watching the situation in Asia and Europe very closely and are preparing for the possibility that the virus may begin to spread more easily and widely from person to person.

Symptoms

Symptoms of avian flu in humans have ranged from typical human flu-like symptoms (fever, cough, sore throat, and muscle aches) to eye infections, pneumonia, severe respiratory diseases (such as acute respiratory distress), and other severe and life-threatening complications.

Transmission

During an outbreak of bird flu among poultry, there is a possible risk to people who have contact with infected birds or surfaces that have been contaminated with secretions or excretions from infected birds.

You cannot get avian influenza from properly handled and cooked poultry and eggs. There currently is no scientific evidence that people have been infected with bird flu by eating safely handled and properly cooked poultry or eggs.

Most cases of avian influenza infection in humans have resulted from direct or close contact with infected poultry or surfaces contaminated with secretions and excretions from infected birds. Even if poultry and eggs were to be contaminated with the virus, proper cooking would kill it. In fact, recent studies have shown that the cooking methods that are already recommended by the U.S. Department of Agriculture (USDA) and the Food and Drug Administration (FDA) for poultry and eggs, to prevent other infections, will destroy influenza viruses as well.

Transmission of Bird Flu Between Animals and People
Influenza A viruses have infected many different animals including ducks, chickens, pigs, whales, horses, and seals. However, certain subtypes of influenza A virus are specific to certain species, except for birds, which are hosts to all known subtypes of influenza A.

Influenza A viruses normally seen in one species sometimes can cross over and cause illness in another species. For example, until 1998, only H1N1 viruses circulated widely in the U.S. pig population. However, in 1998, H3N2 viruses from humans were introduced into the pig population and caused widespread disease among pigs. Later, H3N8 viruses from horses have crossed over and caused outbreaks in dogs, and most recently, the H1N1 virus circulating in the pig population has crossed over to cause illnesses in humans.

Avian influenza A viruses may be transmitted from animals to humans in two main ways:
- Directly from birds or from avian virus-contaminated environments to people.
- Through an intermediate host, such as a pig.

Importing Birds
The U.S. government has determined that there is a risk to importing pet birds from countries experiencing outbreaks of H5N1 avian flu. The CDC and USDA have both taken action to ban the importation of birds from areas where the viurs has been documented.

Bird Feeders

There is no evidence of avian flu having caused disease in birds or people in the United States. At the present time, there is no risk of becoming infected with H5N1 virus from bird feeders. Generally, perching birds (Passeriformes) are the predominate type of birds at feeders. While there are documented cases of avian flu causing death in some Passeriformes (e.g., house sparrow, Eurasian tree-sparrow, house finch), in both free-ranging and experimental settings, none occurred in the U.S. And most of the wild birds that are traditionally associated with avian influenza viruses are waterfowl and shore birds.

Diagnosing Bird Flu

Avian influenza cannot be diagnosed by symptoms alone, so a laboratory test is required. Avian flu is usually diagnosed by collecting a swab from the nose or throat during the first few days of illness. This swab is then sent to a lab, where they will either look for avian influenza virus using a molecular test, or they will try to grow the virus. Growing avian flu viruses should only be done in laboratories with high levels of protection.

If it is late in the illness, it may be difficult to find an avian flu virus directly using these methods. If this is the case, it may still be possible to diagnose avian influenza by looking for evidence of the body's response to the virus. This is not always an option because it requires two blood specimens (one taken during the first few days of illness and another taken some weeks later), and it can take several weeks to verify the results.

Treatment

Studies done in laboratories suggest that some of the prescription medicines approved in the United States for human influenza viruses should work in treating avian influenza infection in humans. However, this evidence is inconclusive and influenza viruses can become resistant to drugs, so even if these medications prove to be effective now, they may not always work. Additional studies are needed to demonstrate the effectiveness of these medicines.

The bird flu that has caused human illness and death in Asia is resistant to amantadine and rimantadine, two antiviral medications commonly used for influenza. Two other antiviral medications, Tamiflu and Relenza, would probably work to treat influenza caused by the virus, but additional studies still need to be done to demonstrate their effectiveness.

A small number of Tamiflu resistant bird flu virus infections have been reported. Efforts to produce pre-pandemic vaccine candidates for humans that would be effective against avian flu viruses are ongoing. However, no vaccines are currently available for human use.

Prevention

The seasonal flu vaccine, commonly administered in doctor's offices and pharmacies, does not provide protection against avian flu. Currently, wearing a mask is not recommended for routine use (e.g., in public) for preventing influenza exposure. In the United States, disposable surgical and procedure masks have been widely used in health-care settings to prevent exposure to respiratory infections, but the masks have not been used commonly in community settings, such as schools, businesses, and public gatherings.

On April 17, 2007, the U.S. Food and Drug Administration announced its approval of the first vaccine to prevent human infection with one strain of the virus. The federal government for the U.S. Strategic National Stockpile has purchased the vaccine, produced by Sanofi Pasteur; it will be distributed by public-health officials if needed. This vaccine will not be made commercially available to the general public.

Other bird flu vaccines are being developed by other companies against different flu strains.

The Sanofi Pasteur vaccine was developed as a safeguard against the possible emergence of a bird flu pandemic. However, the virus is not a pandemic virus because it does not transmit efficiently from person to person, so the vaccine is being held in stockpiles rather than being used by the general public. This vaccine aids preparedness efforts in case a bird flu pandemic were to emerge.

Persons who work with poultry or respond to avian influenza outbreaks among poultry, and are therefore potentially exposed to infected or potentially infected poultry, are advised to follow recommended bio-security and infection control practices including careful attention to hand hygiene and use of appropriate personal protective equipment. In addition, poultry outbreak responders should adhere to guidance from the CDC and WHO, receive seasonal flu vaccinations, and take preventative antiviral medication during an outbreak control response. Seasonal flu vaccines will not prevent infection. Exposed persons should be carefully monitored for symptoms that develop during and in seven days after their last exposure to infected poultry or to environments potentially contaminated with virus excretions/ secretions.

To stay safe, the advice is the same for protecting against any infection from poultry:

- Wash your hands with soap and warm water for at least twenty seconds before and after handling raw poultry and eggs.
- Clean cutting boards and other utensils with soap and hot water to keep raw poultry from contaminating other foods.
- Use a food thermometer to make sure you cook poultry to a temperature of at least 165 degrees Fahrenheit.
- Cook eggs until whites and yolks are firm.

Avian Flu in Animals

Infected birds shed the flu virus in their saliva, nasal secretions, and feces. Susceptible birds become infected when they have contact with contaminated secretions or excretions or with surfaces contaminated by infected birds. Domesticated birds may become infected through direct contact with infected waterfowl or other infected poultry, or through contact with surfaces (such as dirt or cages) or materials (such as water or feed) that have been contaminated with the virus.

Infection in domestic poultry causes two main forms of disease that are distinguished by low and high extremes of virulence. The "low pathogenic" form may go undetected and usually causes only mild symptoms (such as ruffled feathers and a drop in egg production). However, the highly pathogenic form spreads more rapidly through flocks of poultry. This form may cause disease that affects multiple internal organs and has a mortality rate that can reach 90-100%, often within 48 hours.

In addition to humans and birds, we know that pigs, tigers, leopards, ferrets, and domestic cats can be infected with avian flu.

Avian flu is caused by bird flu viruses. These viruses occur naturally among birds. Wild birds worldwide carry the viruses in their intestines, but usually do not get sick from them. However, these viruses are very contagious among birds and can make some domesticated birds, including chickens, ducks, and turkeys very sick and kill them.

Spread of Avian Influenza Viruses among Birds

Avian influenza viruses circulate among birds worldwide. Certain birds, particularly water birds, act as hosts for influenza viruses by carrying the virus in their intestines and shedding it. Infected birds shed virus in saliva, nasal secretions, and feces. Susceptible birds can become infected with avian influenza virus when they have contact with contaminated nasal, respiratory, or fecal material from infected birds. Fecal-to-oral transmission is the most common mode of spread between birds.

Most often, the wild birds that are host to the virus do not get sick, but they can spread it to other birds. Infection with certain viruses can cause widespread disease and death among some species of domesticated birds.

Avian Influenza Outbreaks in Poultry

Avian influenza outbreaks among poultry occur worldwide from time to time. Since 1997, for example, the United States has experienced seventeen incidents of H5 and H7 low pathogenic avian influenza, and one incident of highly pathogenic avian influenza that was restricted to one poultry farm. The U.S. Department of Agriculture monitored and responded to these incidents.

In 2004, the United States experienced the first highly pathogenic avian flu outbreak among poultry in twenty years. The outbreak was reported in a flock of 7,000 chickens in south-central Texas. There was no report of transmission to humans.

People, vehicles, and other inanimate objects such as cages can be vectors for the spread of influenza virus from one farm to another. When this happens, avian influenza outbreaks can occur among poultry.

When highly pathogenic flu viruses cause outbreaks, between 90% and 100% of poultry can die from the infection. Therefore, when outbreaks occur in poultry, quarantine and depopulation (or culling) and surveillance around affected flocks is the preferred control and eradication option.

Domestic Cats and Avian Flu
While domestic cats are not usually susceptible to influenza type A infection, it is known that they can become infected and die from avian flu. All of the cases in domestic cats reported to date have been associated with bird flu outbreaks among domestic poultry or wild birds and are thought to have occurred by the cat eating raw infected birds.

During the avian flu outbreak that occurred from 2003 to 2004 in Asia, there were several unofficial reports of fatal infections in domestic cats. Studies carried out in the Netherlands, and published in 2004, showed that housecats could be infected with avian flu and could spread the virus to other housecats. In these experiments, the cats became sick after direct inoculation of virus isolated from a fatal human case, and following the feeding of infected raw chicken.

As long as there is no avian flu outbreak in the United States, there is no risk of a U.S. cat becoming infected with this disease. The virus circulating in Asia, Europe, and Africa has not yet entered the United States. The CDC is working closely with domestic and international partners to continually monitor this situation.

Wild Cats and Avian Flu

Large cats kept in captivity have been diagnosed with avian flu as well. In December 2003, two tigers and two leopards that were fed fresh chicken carcasses from a local slaughterhouse died at a zoo in Thailand. An investigation identified avian flu as the culprit.

In February and March 2004, the virus was detected in a leopard and a tiger, both of which died in a zoo near Bangkok. In October 2004, 147 of 441 captive tigers in a zoo in Thailand died or were euthanatized as a result of infection after being fed fresh chicken carcasses. The cats are thought to have gotten sick from eating infected raw meat. Results of a subsequent investigation suggested that at least some tiger-to-tiger transmission occurred in that facility.

There is no evidence to date that cats can spread the virus to humans. No cases of avian flu in humans have been linked to exposure to sick cats, and no outbreaks among populations of cats have been reported. All of the infections in cats appear to have been associated with outbreaks in domestic or wild birds and acquired through ingestion of raw meat from an infected bird.

Dogs and Avian Flu
While dogs are not usually susceptible to avian flu viruses, the virus that emerged in Asia in 2003 has been documented to infect other carnivore species (e.g. cats, tigers, leopards, stone martens). This has raised concern that this strain of the virus may be capable of infecting dogs. An unpublished study carried out in 2005 by the National Institute of Animal Health in Bangkok indicated that dogs could be infected with the virus, but no associated disease was detected. This limited information is not enough to determine whether or not dogs are susceptible to the virus.

There is not enough information available about avian flu infection in dogs to know how infection would occur. Affected domestic cats in Europe appear to have become infected by feeding upon raw infected poultry or wild birds. If dogs are susceptible to avian flu, infection may be by the same route.

What is Being Done

There is currently a ban on the importation of birds and bird products from affected countries. The regulation states that no person may import or attempt to import any birds (Class Aves), whether dead or alive, or any products derived from birds (including hatching eggs), from the specified countries.

This prohibition does not apply to any person who imports or attempts to import products derived from birds if, as determined by federal officials, such products have been properly processed to render them noninfectious so that they pose no risk of transmitting or carrying the virus and which comply with the U.S. Department of Agriculture (USDA) requirements. Therefore, feathers from these countries are banned unless they have been processed to render them noninfectious.

In February 2004, the CDC provided U.S. public health departments with recommendations for enhanced surveillance (detection) of H5N1 influenza in the country. Follow-up messages, distributed via the Health Alert Network, were sent to the health departments on August 12, 2004, February 4, 2005, and June 7, 2006; all three notices reminded public health departments about recommendations for detecting, diagnosing, and preventing the spread of the virus. The notices also recommended measures for laboratory testing for the virus.

The CDC is working with WHO and other international partners to monitor the situation closely. In addition, the CDC continues to work with WHO and the National Institutes of Health (NIH) on development of a vaccine.

Common Questions

What are the implications to human health?
Two main risks for human health from avian flu are:
- The risk of direct infection when the virus passes from the infected bird to humans, sometimes resulting in severe disease
- The risk that the virus will change into a form that is highly infectious for humans and spreads easily from person to person, much like what has happened with the H1N1 swine flu virus.

Is it safe to keep a small flock of chickens?
Yes. In the United States there is no need, at present, to remove a flock of chickens because of concerns regarding avian flu. The U.S. Department of Agriculture monitors potential infection of poultry and poultry products.

What are the risks to humans from the recent outbreak?
The avian flu does not usually infect people, but since November 2003, nearly 400 cases of human infection with highly infective avian flu viruses have been reported by more than a dozen countries. This virus has never been detected among wild birds, domestic poultry, or people in the United States. Most of these cases have occurred from direct or close contact with infected poultry or contaminated surfaces; however, a few cases of human-to-human spread have occurred.

Does the CDC recommend travel restrictions?

The CDC does not recommend any travel restrictions to affected countries at this time. However, the CDC currently advises that travelers to countries with known outbreaks avoid poultry farms, contact with animals in live food markets, and any surfaces that appear to be contaminated with feces from poultry or other animals.

6

MRSA

MRSA, discovered in 1961, stands for Methicillin-resistant *Staphylococcus aureus*. MRSA has been called the flesh eating bacteria, and in recent years, has killed more Americans than AIDS has. About 94,000 Americans are infected with MRSA each year. MRSA poses a particularly dangerous problem because antibiotics are not effective, allowing the disease to spread and strengthen in the victims it infects.

Staphylococcus aureus, often referred to simply as "staph," is a bacteria commonly found on the skin and in the nose of healthy people. Occasionally, staphylococci can get into the body and cause an infection. This infection can be minor (such as pimples, boils, and other skin conditions), but has been known to cause conditions such as life threatening pneumonia and necrotized skin and wound infections.

Staph. aureus is a common organism and can be found in the nostrils of up to 30% of persons. Person-to-person transmission is the usual form of spread and occurs through contact with secretions from infected skin lesions, nasal discharge, or spread via the hands.

Due in part to the over-use of antibiotics, MRSA is a staph infection that has developed a resistance to commonly used antibiotics that were previously used to treat such infections. MRSA germs have a unique gene that causes them to be unaffected by all but the highest concentrations of these antibiotics. Therefore, alternate antibiotics must be used to treat persons infected with MRSA. Vancomycin has been the most effective and reliable drug in these cases, but is used intravenously and is not effective for treatment of MRSA when taken by mouth.

Recently, reports have shown that MRSA appears to be spreading among pigs, and research indicates that the bacterial infection can be passed between pigs and humans.

The increasing frequency of antimicrobial resistance is of great concern to both medical providers and the general public. Of particular concern is the possibility of spread of multi-drug resistant germs in the community.

MRSA occurs most frequently among patients who undergo invasive medical procedures or who have weakened immune systems and are being treated in hospitals and healthcare facilities, such as nursing homes and dialysis centers. MRSA, in healthcare settings, commonly causes serious and potentially life threatening infections, such as bloodstream infections, surgical site infections, or pneumonia.

Community infections, reportedly occur in otherwise healthy, non-hospitalized persons without contact with healthcare personnel or other colonized patients. A report of MRSA infections leading to four deaths in previously healthy children demonstrated that MRSA infections can be community-acquired in persons with no exposure to the hospital system. This raises serious concerns about the possibility of transmission of MRSA outside the healthcare system. If MRSA becomes the most common form of *Staphylococcus aureus* in a community, it will make treatment of common infections much more difficult.

MRSA is a dangerous type of staph bacteria that is not only resistant to antibiotics, but may also cause other types of infections. As with all regular staph infections, recognizing the signs and receiving treatment for MRSA in the early stages reduces the chances of the infection becoming severe.

Most MRSA skin infections appear as pustules or boils which often are red, swollen, painful, or have pus or other drainage. These skin infections commonly occur at sites of visible skin trauma, such as cuts and abrasions, and areas of the body covered by hair (back of neck, groin, buttock, armpit, beard area of men).

The main mode of transmission to other patients is through human hands, especially healthcare workers' hands. Hands may become contaminated with MRSA bacteria by contact with infected or colonized patients. If appropriate hand hygiene such as washing with soap and water or using an alcohol-based hand sanitizer is not performed, the bacteria can be spread when the healthcare worker touches other patients.

Along with MRSA, many significant infection-causing bacteria in the world are becoming resistant to the most commonly prescribed antimicrobial treatments. What causes this and what does it mean?

Antibiotic or antimicrobial resistance occurs when bacteria change or adapt in a way that allows them to survive in the presence of antibiotics designed to kill them. In some cases, bacteria become so resistant that no available antibiotics are effective against them. At this time, treatment options still exist for healthcare-associated MRSA.

People infected with antibiotic-resistant organisms like MRSA are more likely to have longer and more expensive hospital stays, and may be more likely to die as a result of the infection. When the drug of choice for treating their infection doesn't work, they require treatment with second or third choice medicines that may be less effective, more toxic, and more expensive.

MRSA is becoming more prevalent in healthcare settings. According to CDC data, the proportion of infections that are resistant to antibiotics has been growing. In 1974, MRSA infections accounted for two percent of the total number of staph infections; in 1995 it was 22%; in 2004 it was 63%. Of the MRSA infections contracted in the hospital, 20% of them result in death.

Symptoms

Most staph skin infections, including MRSA, appear as a bump or infected area on the skin that may be:
- Red
- Swollen
- Painful
- Warm to the touch
- Full of pus or other drainage
- Accompanied by a fever

Transmission

In the case of MRSA, patients who already have MRSA infection or who carry the bacteria on their bodies but do not have symptoms (colonized) are the most common sources of transmission.

MRSA is usually transmitted by direct skin-to-skin contact or contact with shared items or surfaces that have come into contact with someone else's infection (towels and used bandages). Though MRSA skin infections can occur anywhere, some settings have factors that make it easier for MRSA to be transmitted. These factors, referred to as the five C's, are as follows:

> Crowding
> Contact (frequent skin-to-skin)
> Compromised skin (i.e., cuts or abrasions)
> Contaminated items and surfaces
> Cleanliness (lack of)

Locations where the five C's are common include schools, dormitories, military barracks, households, correctional facilities, and daycare centers. MRSA is spread by:

- Having direct contact with another person's infection
- Sharing personal items, such as towels or razors, that have touched infected skin
- Touching surfaces or items, such as used bandages, contaminated with MRSA

MRSA has been found to live in steam baths; both in the inside seating area and outside bench areas. Cleaning the seating areas with a dilute bleach solution after use appears to be the most effective way to disinfect steam baths. Also, a barrier to prevent direct contact with the seat (such as cardboard) may be a way to prevent spread of MRSA in the steam bath. More research needs to be done to determine how effective these methods are for preventing illness.

The role of the environment in the spread of staph and MRSA in community settings is unclear. These infections are most often found on people and not naturally found in the environment. Staph and MRSA could get into the environment if your hands can pick them up by touching infected skin or certain areas of the body where these bacteria can live (like the nose). Then, if you touch a surface or item like a towel, your hands can pass the bacteria on to these items you have touched.

Even if surfaces have staph and MRSA on them, this does not mean that you will definitely get an infection if you touch those surfaces. Staph and MRSA are most likely to cause problems when you have a cut or scrape that is not covered. That's why it's important to cover your cuts and open wounds with bandages. MRSA can also get into small openings in the skin, like the openings at hair follicles. The best defense is good hygiene. Keep your hands clean, use a barrier like clothing or towels between you and any surfaces you share with others (like gym equipment), and shower immediately after activities that involve direct skin contact with others. These are easy ways to decrease your risk of getting a staph or MRSA infection.

As with other germs, staph and MRSA can survive on some surfaces for hours, days, or even months, but it all depends on factors like temperature, humidity, the amount of germs present, and the type of surface (is it porous like a sponge or nonporous like plastic?). It also depends on whether these surfaces have nutrients to allow it to survive longer. When surfaces aren't cleaned and conditions are good for bacterial growth, staph and MRSA is more likely to survive for longer periods.

Global Time Bomb

Diagnosing MRSA

MRSA cannot be diagnosed just by looking at the infection site. Many start out as minor looking scrapes or cuts and worsen over time. Doctors often diagnose MRSA by checking a tissue sample or nasal secretions for signs of drug-resistant bacteria. Current diagnostic procedures involve sending a sample to a lab where it is placed in a dish of nutrients that encourage bacterial growth (a culture). It takes about 48 hours for the bacteria to grow. However, newer tests that can detect staph DNA in a matter of hours are becoming more widely available. This will help healthcare providers decide on the proper treatment regimen for a patient more quickly, after an official diagnosis has been made.

In the hospital, you might be tested for MRSA if you show signs of infection, or if you are transferred to a hospital from another healthcare setting where MRSA is known to be present. You also might be tested if you have had a previous history of MRSA.

Treatment

When MRSA skin infections occur, cleaning and disinfection should be performed on surfaces that are likely to contact uncovered or poorly covered infections. Cleaning surfaces with detergent-based cleaners or Environmental Protection Agency (EPA) registered disinfectants is effective at removing MRSA from the environment.

If you suspect you may have a MRSA skin infection, cover the area with a bandage and contact your healthcare professional. It is especially important to contact your healthcare professional if signs and symptoms are accompanied by a fever.

Almost all MRSA skin infections can be effectively treated by drainage of pus with or without antibiotics. More serious infections, such as pneumonia, bloodstream infections, or bone infections, are very rare in healthy people.

Treatment for aggressive MRSA may include having a healthcare professional drain the infection and, in some cases, prescribe an antibiotic. Do not attempt to drain the infection yourself—doing so could worsen or spread it to others. If you are given an antibiotic, be sure to take all of the doses (even if the infection is getting better), unless your healthcare professional tells you to stop taking it.

The antibiotics most likely to work against a resistant MRSA infection include Bactrim, Cleocin, Cubicin, Synercid, Vancocin, and Zyvox. Some of these can only be administered intravenously, and resistance is already being seen with some of these medications.

Prevention

A possible vaccine has been developed and has shown promise for preventing the most serious MRSA infections in mice, rabbits, monkeys, and in one high risk group, dialysis patients. However, this has not been tested in otherwise healthy persons. This vaccine has not been approved by the FDA and approval will require further evidence of effectiveness.

If you have a MRSA skin infection, cover your wound. Keep wounds that are draining or have pus covered with clean, dry bandages until healed. Follow your healthcare provider's instructions on proper care of the wound. Pus from infected wounds can contain staph, including MRSA, so keeping the infection covered will help prevent the possible spread to others. Bandages and tape can be discarded with the regular trash.

Clean your hands frequently. You, your family, and others in close contact should wash their hands frequently with soap and water or use an alcohol-based hand sanitizer, especially after changing the bandage or touching the infected wound.

Avoid sharing personal items, such as towels, washcloths, razors, clothing, or uniforms, that may have had contact with the infected wound or bandage. Wash sheets, towels, and clothes that become soiled with water and laundry detergent. Use a dryer to dry clothes completely.

During a MRSA outbreak in Alaska, prior use of antibiotics was found to be a risk factor for MRSA infection. Therefore, the appropriate use of antibiotics is recommended (i.e., use only when needed to treat bacterial infections) to prevent the development of resistant strains and possibly reduce risk of infection.

Cleaning to Prevent the Spread of MRSA
Focus on surfaces that touch people's bare skin each day and any surfaces that could come into contact with uncovered infections. For example, surfaces such as benches in the weight room or locker room.

Large surfaces such as floors and walls have not been directly involved in the spread of staph and MRSA. There is no evidence that spraying or fogging rooms or surfaces with disinfectants will prevent staph and MRSA infections more effectively than the targeted approach of cleaning frequently touched surfaces and any surfaces that have been exposed to infections.

Cleaners or detergents are products that are used to remove soil, dirt, dust, organic matter, and germs (like bacteria, viruses, and fungi). Cleaners or detergents work by washing the surface to lift dirt and germs off surfaces so they can be rinsed away with water. The same thing happens when you wash your hands with soap and water or when you wash dishes. Rinsing is an important part of the cleaning process.

Sanitizers are used to reduce germs from surfaces but not totally get rid of them. Sanitizers reduce the germs from surfaces to levels that are considered safe.

Disinfectants are chemical products that destroy or inactivate germs and prevent them from growing. Disinfectants have no effect on dirt, soil, or dust. Disinfectants are regulated by the U.S. Environmental Protection Agency (EPA). You can use a disinfectant after cleaning for surfaces that have visible blood or drainage from infected skin.

Effective Disinfectants

Disinfectants effective against *Staphylococcus aureus* or staph are most likely also effective against MRSA. These products are readily available from grocery stores and other retail stores. Check the disinfectant product's label on the back of the container. Most, if not all, disinfectant manufacturers will provide a list of germs on the label that the product can destroy. Use disinfectants that are registered by the EPA (check for an EPA registration number on the product's label to confirm that it is registered).

Read the label first. Each cleaner and disinfectant has instructions on the label that tell you important facts:
- How to apply the product to a surface.
- How long you need to leave it on the surface to be effective (contact time).
- If the surface needs to be cleaned first and rinsed after using.

- If the disinfectant is safe for the surface.
- Whether the product requires dilution with water before use.
- Precautions you should take when applying the product such wearing gloves or aprons or making sure you have good ventilation during application.

Contact time is the time needed for the disinfectant to inactivate or kill germs to the extent as indicated by the manufacturer. For example, if a disinfectant label says that the product will inactivate 99.99% of germs, and the contact time of 1 minute is in the instructions, this means that this disinfectant will inactivate or kill 99.99% of germs in one minute *if you follow the instructions.* Most instructions will note that the disinfectant must remain wet on the pre-cleaned surface being treated for the entire contact time in order to be effective.

Some surfaces need to be cleaned before being disinfected, so read the label first. Soil, dirt, dust, and organic matter all can often interfere with the active ingredients of disinfectants. Removing dirt from a surface by cleaning the surface before using a disinfectant will make sure it is most effective. Follow the product label's instructions. Most products will use the words "pre-cleaned surface" to point out that a surface should be cleaned before using the disinfectant.

Some disinfectants can be respiratory, eye and/or skin irritants. Read and follow the product label instructions. The product label is your guide to using disinfectants safely and effectively. It contains information that you should read and understand before you use the product.

Many items such as computer keyboards or handheld electronic devices may be difficult to clean or disinfect or they could be damaged if they became wet. If these items are touched by many people during the course of the day, a cleanable cover/skin could be used on the item to allow for cleaning while protecting the item. Always check to see if the manufacturer has instructions for cleaning.

Although in most situations you will not know if a surface has been cleaned, it's important to remember that most surfaces do not pose a risk of spreading staph and MRSA.

Chlorine Bleach as a Disinfectant

In general, EPA-registered products are preferred for disinfection, but if these aren't available, household chlorine bleach can be used. Chlorine bleach is a broad spectrum disinfectant that can inactivate or kill germs, including staph and MRSA. It should never be used at full strength for disinfecting. If you are using household chlorine bleach, read the label to see if the product has specific instructions for disinfection. Some bleach products are EPA-registered for this purpose.

If no disinfection instructions exist, then use 1/4 cup of regular household bleach in 1 gallon of water (a 1:100 dilution equivalent) to disinfect pre-cleaned surfaces. As with other cleaners and disinfectants, household chlorine bleach might damage some surfaces and items—for instance, some metals, plastics, and non-colorfast clothing.

Also be aware that household chlorine bleach, like other disinfectants, can be skin, eye, and respiratory irritants. Take appropriate precautions described on the product's label instructions to reduce this risk. You might need to wear protective gear such as gloves.

Never mix chlorine bleach with any other household or cleaning products. Doing so can result in different types of harmful acids and gases. Disinfectants are registered by the EPA as pesticides and are not to be used on skin or other body parts, and are thus inappropriate for treating MRSA skin infections.

Routine Laundry

Routine laundry procedures, detergents, and laundry additives will all help to make clothes, towels, and linens safe to wear or touch. If items have been contaminated by infectious material, these may be laundered separately, but this is not absolutely necessary.

Read and follow the clothing and soap or detergent label instructions. Water temperatures for household laundry depend on the type of fiber or fabric of the clothing. In general, wash and dry in the warmest temperatures recommended on the clothing label. In addition, some modern laundry detergents are made to clean best at certain temperatures. Not following instructions could damage the clothing item or decrease the effectiveness of the detergent. Hot water washing is not necessary for all household laundry.

The use of bleach is not necessary for routine laundry loads. Clean laundry produced by washing with detergent alone will be safe for wear and use. Use of bleach as a disinfectant in laundering is optional, and not all fabrics are suitable for bleach. Read the clothing label instructions.

MRSA and Schools

The decision to close a school for any communicable disease should be made by school officials in consultation with local and/or state public health officials. However, in most cases, it is not necessary to close schools because of a MRSA infection in a student. It is important to note that MRSA transmission can be prevented by simple measures such as hand hygiene and covering infections.

Covering infections will greatly reduce the risks of surfaces becoming contaminated. In general, it is not necessary to close schools to "disinfect" them when MRSA infections occur. MRSA is transmitted primarily by skin-to-skin contact and contact with surfaces that have come into contact with someone else's infection.

Usually, it should not be necessary to inform the entire school community about a single MRSA infection. When an MRSA infection occurs within the school population, the school nurse and school physician should determine, based on their medical judgment, whether some or all students, parents, and staff should be notified. Consultation with the local public health authorities should be used to guide this decision.

Remember that staphylococcus (staph) bacteria, including MRSA, have been and remain a common cause of skin infections. Consult with your school about its policy for notification of skin infections. Unless directed by a physician, students with MRSA infections should not be excluded from attending school.

Teachers and School Personnel:
- If you observe children with open draining wounds or infections, refer the child to the school nurse.
- Enforce hand hygiene with soap and water or alcohol-based hand sanitizers (if available) before eating and after using the bathroom.
- Students with skin infections may need to be referred to a licensed health care provider for diagnosis and treatment. School health personnel should notify parents/guardians when possible skin infections are detected.

Global Time Bomb

- Use standard precautions (e.g., hand hygiene before and after contact, wearing gloves) when caring for non-intact skin or potential infections.
- Use barriers such as gowns, masks, and eye protection if splashing of body fluids is anticipated.

Athletic Directors and Coaches

- Athletic facilities such as locker rooms should always be kept clean whether or not MRSA infections have occurred among the athletes.
- Review cleaning procedures and schedules with the janitorial/environmental service staff.
- Cleaning procedures should focus on commonly touched surfaces and surfaces that come into direct contact with people's bare skin each day.
- Cleaning with detergent-based cleaners or EPA registered detergents/disinfectants will remove MRSA from surfaces.
- Cleaners and disinfectants, including household chlorine bleach, can be irritating and exposure to these chemicals has been associated with health problems such as asthma and skin and eye irritation.
- Take appropriate precautions described on the product's label instructions to reduce exposure. Wearing personal protective equipment such as gloves and eye protection may be indicated.
- Follow the instruction labels on all cleaners and disinfectants, including household chlorine bleach, to make sure they are used safely and correctly.

Cleaning Sports Equipment

Equipment, such as helmets and protective gear, should be cleaned according to the equipment manufacturers' instructions to make sure the cleaner will not harm the item. Shared equipment should be cleaned after each use and allowed to dry.

Excluding Athletes with MRSA

If sport-specific rules do not exist, in general, athletes should be excluded if wounds cannot be properly covered during participation. The phrase "properly covered" means that the skin infection is covered by a securely attached bandage or dressing that will contain all drainage and will remain intact throughout the activity. If wounds can be properly covered, good hygiene measures should be stressed to the athlete such as performing hand hygiene before and after changing bandages and throwing used bandages in the trash.

A healthcare provider might exclude an athlete if the activity poses a risk to the health of the infected athlete (such as injury to the infected area), even though the infection can be properly covered. Athletes with active infections or open wounds should not use whirlpools or therapy pools not cleaned between athletes and other common-use water facilities like swimming pools until infections and wounds are healed.

If you notice an athlete with a possible infection:
- Refer athletes with possible infections to a healthcare provider such as team physician, athletic trainer, school nurse, or primary care doctor.
- If the athlete is less than 18 years old, notify parents/guardians of the athlete about the possible infection.
- Educate athletes on ways to prevent spreading the infection.
- Using the criteria above, consider excluding the athlete from participation until evaluated by a healthcare provider.

Improve Hygiene

Make sure supplies are available to comply with prevention measures (soap in shower and at sinks, bandages for covering wounds, hand hygiene such as alcohol-based hand rubs).

Enforce policies and encourage practices designed to prevent disease spread. Make sure athletes:

- o keep wounds covered and contained
- o shower immediately after participation
- o shower before using whirlpools
- o wash and dry uniforms after each use

For Medical Personnel

When a patient has a skin infection, it may very likely be MRSA. Recent data suggest that MRSA in the community is increasing. The spectrum of disease caused by MRSA appears to be similar to that of *Staphylococcus aureus* in the community. Skin and soft tissue infections (SSTIs), specifically furuncles (abscessed hair follicles or "boils"), carbuncles (coalesced masses of furuncles), and abscesses, are the most frequently reported clinical manifestations. The role of MRSA in cellulitis without abscess or purulent drainage is less clear since cultures are rarely obtained.

When to Consider MRSA

The Centers for Disease Control and Prevention encourages you to consider MRSA in the differential diagnosis of SSTIs compatible with *S. aureus* infections, especially those that are purulent (fluctuant or palpable fluid-filled cavity, yellow or white center, central point or "head," draining pus, or possible to aspirate pus with needle or syringe). A patient's presenting complaint of "spider bite" should raise suspicion of a S. aureus infection.

Primary Treatment Options for MRSA Skin Infections

Incision and drainage constitutes the primary therapy for these purulent skin infections. Empiric antimicrobial coverage for MRSA may be warranted in addition to incision and drainage based on clinical assessment (presence of systemic symptoms, severe local symptoms, immune suppression, extremes of patient age, infections in a difficult to drain area, or lack of response to incision and drainage alone). For severe infections, consider consulting with an infectious disease specialist. Obtaining specimens for culture and susceptibility testing is useful to guide therapy, particularly for those who fail to respond adequately to initial management.

MRSA skin infections can develop into more serious infections. It is important to discuss a follow-up plan with your patients in case they develop systemic symptoms or worsening local symptoms, or if symptoms do not improve within 48 hours.

Educate Patients to Prevent Spread

Patient education is a critical component of MRSA case management. Healthcare professionals should educate patients, caretakers and, when possible, household members on methods to avoid MRSA transmission to close contacts.

Appendix A

Instances of Avian Flu Infections in Humans

Confirmed instances of avian influenza A virus infections of humans since 1996 include:

- **United Kingdom, 1996**: One adult developed an eye infection after a piece of straw contacted her eye while cleaning a duck house. Avian flu was detected in the eye fluid sample. The person was not hospitalized and recovered.

- **Hong Kong, 1997**: Highly infective infections occurred in both poultry and humans. This was the first time an avian influenza A virus transmission directly from birds to humans had been found to cause respiratory illness. During this outbreak, eighteen people were hospitalized and six of them died. To control the outbreak, authorities culled about 1.5 million chickens to remove the source of the virus. The most significant risk factor for human illness was visiting a live poultry market in the week before illness onset.

- **China and Hong Kong, 1999**: A less infective avian flu was confirmed in two hospitalized children and resulted in uncomplicated influenza-like illness. Both patients recovered, and no additional cases were confirmed.

- **Virginia, 2002**: Following an outbreak among poultry in the Shenandoah Valley poultry production area, one person developed uncomplicated influenza-like illness.

- **China and Hong Kong, 2003**: Two cases of highly infective avian flu occurred among members of a Hong Kong family that had traveled to China. One person recovered, the other died. How or where these two family members were infected was not determined. Another family member died of a respiratory illness in China, but no testing was done to determine the cause of death.

- **Netherlands, 2003**: The Netherlands reported outbreaks of highly infective avian flu viruses among poultry on multiple farms. Overall, 89 people were confirmed to have infections associated with poultry outbreaks. Most human cases occurred among poultry workers.

  Illness was generally mild and included 78 cases of eye infections; five cases of eye infections combined with influenza-like illness of fever, cough, and muscle aches; two cases of flu-like illness; and four cases that were classified as "other." One death occurred in a veterinarian who visited one of the affected farms and developed complications from infection, including acute respiratory distress syndrome.

  The majority of cases occurred through direct contact with infected poultry. However, Dutch authorities reported three possible instances of human-to-human transmission from poultry workers to family members.

- **Hong Kong, 2003**: Infection was confirmed in a child in Hong Kong. The child was hospitalized with flu-like illness and recovered.

- **New York, 2003**: In November 2003, a patient with serious pre-existing medical conditions was admitted to a hospital in New York with respiratory symptoms. The patient recovered and went home after a few weeks. Testing revealed that the patient had been infected with a avian flu; the patient's underlying medical conditions likely contributed to the severity of the patient's illness.

- **Canada, 2004:** In March 2004, two poultry workers who were assisting in culling operations during a large poultry outbreak had eye infections, one of whom also had a head cold. Both poultry workers recovered. One worker was infected with less infective virus and the other with highly infective virus.

- **China, Thailand, and Vietnam, 2003-2004:** In late 2003 and early 2004, severe and fatal human infections were associated with widespread poultry outbreaks. Most cases had pneumonia and many had respiratory failure. Additional human cases were reported during mid-2004, and late 2004. Most cases appeared to be associated with direct contact with sick or dead poultry. One instance of possible, limited human-to-human spread is believed to have occurred in Thailand. Overall, fifty human cases with thirty-six deaths were reported from three countries.

- **Cambodia, China, Indonesia, Thailand, Vietnam, 2005:** Severe and fatal human infections were associated with the ongoing infections among poultry in the region. Overall, ninety-eight human cases with forty-three deaths were reported from five countries.

- **Azerbaijan, Cambodia, China, Djibouti, Egypt, Indonesia, Iraq, Thailand, Turkey, 2006:** Severe and fatal human infections occurred in association with the ongoing and expanding poultry infections. While most of these cases occurred as a result of contact with infected poultry, in Azerbaijan, the most plausible cause of human exposure is thought to be contact with infected swans.

The largest family cluster of cases to date occurred in North Sumatra, Indonesia during May 2006, with seven confirmed cases and one probable case, including seven deaths. Overall, 115 human cases with 79 deaths were reported in nine countries.

- **Cambodia, China, Egypt, Indonesia, Laos, Myanmar, Nigeria, Pakistan, Vietnam, 2007**: Severe and fatal human infections occurred in association with poultry outbreaks. In addition, during 2007, Nigeria, Laos, Myanmar, and Pakistan confirmed their first human infections. Overall, nine countries reported 86 human cases with 59 deaths in 2007.

- **United Kingdom, 2007**: Human infection resulting in flu-like illness and eye infections were identified in four hospitalized cases. The cases were associated with a poultry outbreak in Wales.

- **Hong Kong, 2007**: In March 2007, infection was confirmed in a 9-month-old Hong Kong girl with mild signs of disease.

Appendix B

MRSA in Alaska

Infections due to *S. aureus* have long been common among rural Alaskans. In 1984, a large outbreak of *Staph. aureus* boils occurred in the village of Kotlik. These were due to a methicillin-sensitive strain. However, in 1996, an Alaska community reported an outbreak of boils caused by *S. aureus* in healthy persons. In some of the patients, cultures of revealed MRSA. Steam-bathing, a common practice among some Alaska populations, was associated with infection and especially the practices of bathing without sitting on a towel or use of personal soap. Recent anecdotal reports from clinicians and laboratories in rural and urban Alaska indicate that infections due to MRSA are becoming increasingly common and present significant therapeutic challenges. These reports raise concerns that MRSA infections are more common and widespread that was previously realized.

In August 2000, health care providers in Southwestern Alaska reported an increase in MRSA skin infections among Alaska Natives, many of whom had no previous hospital exposure. By evaluating laboratory and medical records, large outbreaks of community-onset MRSA infections were found to have occurred in Southwestern Alaska during 1999 and 2000. Over 80% of culture-confirmed *S. aureus* infections during this period were MRSA, 84% of MRSA infections involved skin or soft tissue, but more serious or invasive disease was rare.

Unlike a typical hospital-acquired MRSA, isolates from this outbreak were unlikely to be resistant to multiple antimicrobial classes. Patients with MRSA skin infections were more likely to have received an antimicrobial prescription in the 180 days before their infection than were patients with methicillin-susceptible *Staph. aureus* skin infections. Steam bathing was also a factor in this outbreak. MRSA infections were more common among people who used steam baths.